Table of Contents

THE CASTOR OIL BIBLE

Discover the Ancient Secret to Radiant Skin and Lustrous Hair. 120+ Scientifically-Proven Natural Remedies for Youthful Glow, Anti-Aging, and Timeless Beauty.

**Scan the QR code or click the link on the last page of this book
to download your fantastic bonus!**

Introduction

The Promise of Castor Oil: Unlock the Ancient Secret for Radiant Health and Beauty

Have you ever wondered if there's a natural secret to beauty and health that transcends modern skincare and medical treatments? Welcome to "The Castor Oil Bible," a comprehensive guide where ancient wisdom meets modern science in the relentless pursuit of wellness and natural beauty. This book is your gateway to discovering the myriad benefits of castor oil, a time-honored remedy that has been used for thousands of years but is only now gaining the scientific recognition it deserves.

Castor oil, derived from the seeds of the Ricinus communis plant, has been documented throughout history for its powerful healing properties. From the tombs of ancient Egypt to the texts of Greek medicine, castor oil has been revered as a potent healer. However, despite its rich history, only in recent decades have scientific studies begun to acknowledge its benefits in health and beauty contexts.

This book delves into the depths of castor oil's legacy, exploring its numerous applications and the reasons behind its enduring usage. You will learn not just about the oil itself but also how it has been integrated into various cultures and medical systems over the centuries. Each page of "The Castor Oil Bible" reveals its holistic benefits, which include enhancing skin hydration, promoting hair growth, reducing inflammation, and even boosting immune system function.

The resurgence of interest in natural and organic remedies has paved the way for castor oil to become a cornerstone of alternative medicine. With wellness enthusiasts and health practitioners advocating for more natural approaches to health care, castor oil's popularity is rapidly growing. This book harnesses that momentum and provides readers with scientifically-backed, practical uses of castor oil, making it accessible to a modern audience seeking sustainable and effective health and beauty solutions.

By embracing the teachings of "The Castor Oil Bible," you are not just turning to a single natural remedy but opening a door to a world where beauty and well-being are in harmony with nature. This book aims to bridge the gap between ancient remedies and contemporary scientific approaches, offering a balanced perspective on how castor oil can be a key element in achieving a healthier, more vibrant life.

Through engaging narratives and detailed research, "The Castor Oil Bible" invites you to explore the timeless secrets of castor oil. It is not merely a retrospective look at this amazing oil but a comprehensive guide that equips you with the knowledge to utilize its powers fully. Whether you are new to the concept of natural health or a seasoned practitioner, this book will provide you with the insights and tools necessary to transform your approach to health and beauty.

Prepare to be captivated by the rich history and the transformative properties of castor oil. As you turn each page, you will uncover the ways in which this ancient remedy can be adapted to suit modern-day health and beauty needs. "The Castor Oil Bible" is more than just a book; it is a revelation that will enlighten and inspire you to embrace the natural powers of castor oil in your daily life.

Who Should Read This Book?

"The Castor Oil Bible" is meticulously crafted for those who are ready to embark on a journey towards a more natural and sustainable approach to health and beauty. This comprehensive guide is ideal for anyone, whether you're battling with persistent skin problems, suffering from hair loss, experiencing chronic discomfort, or simply seeking to enhance your overall well-being through holistic practices. The insights provided in this book are designed to cater to a wide range of needs, offering practical, easy-to-use remedies that are supported by both time-honored traditions and modern scientific findings.

If you find yourself constantly navigating the aisles of health stores looking for chemical-free alternatives, or if you're spending hours online searching for non-toxic solutions for your family's health needs, then "The Castor Oil Bible" is written specifically for you. It's also perfect for healthcare practitioners who wish to integrate more natural remedies into their treatment plans, providing them with reliable, scientifically-backed applications of castor oil.

This book is a resource for parents who are on the lookout for safe, natural treatments for their children's minor ailments, such as skin rashes or digestive issues. It's equally valuable for athletes seeking natural remedies for inflammation and muscle soreness, as well as older adults looking for effective, non-invasive methods to relieve arthritis and improve joint health. Beauty enthusiasts will also find this book invaluable, as it offers natural, effective solutions to enhance skin and hair health without the harsh effects of commercial products.

Throughout "The Castor Oil Bible," you'll find a variety of applications that go beyond mere health and beauty. This book provides a holistic view of well-being that includes boosting your immune system, enhancing digestion, and promoting emotional balance through the use of castor oil. Each chapter offers detailed, step-by-step guidance on how to prepare and use these remedies effectively, ensuring that readers can easily incorporate them into their daily routines.

Moreover, this guide does not merely suggest castor oil as a panacea; instead, it presents a balanced view of how this ancient oil can play a crucial role in a comprehensive approach to health and wellness. It encourages readers to combine these remedies with a healthy lifestyle and diet for optimal benefits, illustrating how castor oil can complement other health practices and treatments.

For those who are eco-conscious and striving to lead a green, sustainable life, "The Castor Oil Bible" aligns with your values by promoting treatments that are not only good for you but also kind to the planet. This book emphasizes the importance of using organic, high-quality castor oil to ensure the best results without compromising environmental ethics.

Why This Book Was Written

As someone deeply immersed in the world of natural health, I've witnessed the profound impact that holistic remedies can have on one's well-being. My journey with castor oil began out of necessity when conventional treatments and commercial products repeatedly fell short of providing lasting relief. This experience sparked a passion within me to explore and harness the transformative power of natural remedies, especially castor oil, known for its remarkable healing properties. The decision to write "The Castor Oil Bible" stemmed from an urgent need to share this knowledge with others who, like me, have searched for more authentic, sustainable health solutions.

This book is the culmination of years of research, experimentation, and personal experience, aimed at providing a comprehensive guide to one of nature's most versatile oils. It's designed to serve as a practical manual that not only educates but also empowers readers to take control of their health in ways they might not have thought possible. By focusing on castor oil, a remedy that has stood the test of time, this book sheds light on the myriad ways it can be used to promote health, alleviate pain, and enhance beauty.

In writing this book, I aimed to challenge the status quo of modern medicine and beauty industries that often prioritize quick fixes over sustainable health. Our society has become accustomed to solutions that mask symptoms rather than address underlying issues. "The Castor Oil Bible" introduces a different philosophy: one that advocates for prevention, holistic healing, and nurturing the body naturally. It's about rediscovering ancient wisdom and integrating it with modern science to foster wellness at its core.

The book also serves as a response to the growing disillusionment with the adverse effects of pharmaceuticals and the desire for a more organic, less invasive approach to health care. It caters to those who have become skeptical of one-size-fits-all solutions and are looking for alternatives that are gentle yet effective. This guide aims to reintroduce the simplicity and efficacy of using castor oil, showcasing its wide range of applications from treating skin conditions and hair problems to soothing digestive issues and boosting immune function.

Moreover, "The Castor Oil Bible" was written to fill a gap in the available resources about natural health remedies. While there are countless texts on herbal medicine and natural therapies, few provide the level of detail, scientific backing, and practical advice found in this book. It's structured to guide you step-by-step, ensuring that each remedy can be safely and effectively implemented, with tips for sourcing high-quality ingredients and making the most out of each application.

This book is also a call to action, encouraging readers to take an active role in their health management. It's meant to inspire confidence in the ability to use natural remedies, such as castor oil, to not only treat ailments but also to promote a lifestyle that sustains optimal health. By sharing personal anecdotes and success stories, the book connects with readers on a personal level, making the case for natural remedies more compelling and relatable.

Ultimately, "The Castor Oil Bible" represents a journey back to the roots of medicinal practices, where healing was more about balance and harmony with nature than about combating symptoms. This book invites you to explore the rich tapestry of benefits that castor oil offers, making it a must-have for anyone interested in enhancing their health naturally. It's not just about reading; it's about transforming lives through the power of knowledge and nature.

What's Inside: A Comprehensive Guide Across Six Books

This isn't just a book; it's six books rolled into one comprehensive guide on everything castor oil can offer you, each book dedicated to different facets of castor oil's vast benefits:

Book 1: Introduction to Castor Oil

Dive into the rich history and origins of castor oil, from its ancient uses and cultural significance across various civilizations to its enduring impact in modern times.
Understand the science behind castor oil, exploring key components like Ricinoleic Acid and Omega-9 Fatty Acids and their profound effects on skin, hair, and overall health.
Learn about the different types and grades of castor oil available in the market, including Cold-Pressed vs. Refined, Organic, Hexane-Free options, and the differences between Black and Regular Castor Oil.

Book 2: Preparing and Using Castor Oil

Master the safe preparation and application of castor oil with detailed dos and don'ts, how to make castor oil packs for detox and healing, and tips for maintaining freshness.
Experiment with DIY castor oil recipes tailored for beginners, blending castor oil with essential oils, and infusing it with herbs to enhance its benefits.
Integrate castor oil into your daily routines seamlessly, with advice on making it a staple in both morning and evening rituals, quick hacks for busy schedules, and travel-friendly solutions.

Book 3: Castor Oil for Radiant Skin

Achieve clear, glowing skin with techniques like the castor oil cleansing method tailored for acne-prone skin, anti-aging serums, and masks that provide an instant glow.
Address specific skin issues with tailored solutions for eczema, psoriasis, dry skin, as well as scars, stretch marks, and sunburns.
Extend the benefits to your lips, nails, and hands with nourishing balms, strengthening treatments, and hydrating solutions.

Book 4: Castor Oil for Lustrous Hair

Enhance hair growth and thickness with specialized oil blends, scalp massages, and hot oil treatments designed to combat hair loss, thinning, and alopecia.
Maintain healthy, shiny hair through nourishing shampoos, conditioners, hair masks for damage repair and shine, and treatments for split ends and dry scalp.
Care for your eyebrows and eyelashes with growth serums and conditioners, alongside tips for achieving fuller, more defined brows.

Book 5: Castor Oil for Anti-Aging and Timeless Beauty

Prevent premature aging with collagen-boosting serums, eye creams for puffiness and dark circles, and night oils that deeply moisturize.
Discover skin tightening and firming solutions, including neck and décolletage oils, cellulite treatments, and body wraps for toning.
Promote overall wellness and longevity through detoxification, lymphatic drainage, hormonal balance, menopause relief, and vitality-enhancing practices.

Book 6: Castor Oil for Digestive Health and Detox

Utilize castor oil packs for digestive relief, detailing their preparation, uses for IBS, constipation, and bloating, and their role in liver detoxification.
Explore gut healing and inflammation reduction with the castor oil and gut-brain health connection, anti-inflammatory elixirs, and solutions for treating leaky gut syndrome and ulcers.
Support weight loss and metabolism enhancement with castor oil, featuring recipes for metabolism-boosting smoothies and wraps for targeted fat reduction.

In addition to the wealth of knowledge spread across six detailed books in "The Castor Oil Bible," you'll also receive five incredible bonuses. These handpicked bonuses are designed to complement the core content, offering even more ways to enhance your health, beauty, and home environment naturally. Dive into these special additions that ensure you get the most comprehensive guide to utilizing castor oil in all aspects of your life.

Bonus 1: The Castor Oil Manifesto: 120 Recipes for Natural Wellness.
Dive into an extensive collection of castor oil recipes that promise to enhance your health and beauty routines naturally. From soothing balms to rejuvenating serums, each recipe offers a gateway to wellness.

Bonus 2: Unleash Nature's Secret: Boost Your Immunity and Ease Pain Naturally.
Unlock the powerful secrets of castor oil to fortify your immune system and alleviate pain. This guide

provides you with simple, effective techniques to tap into the anti-inflammatory and immune-boosting properties of castor oil.

Bonus 3: Harmonize Your Hormones: Discover Natural Fertility and Wellbeing Solutions.
Explore natural pathways to balance your hormones and enhance fertility with castor oil. This resource offers holistic approaches to hormone health, helping you regain balance and vitality.

Bonus 4: Family Health Redefined: Gentle Remedies for Lifelong Vitality.
Transform your family's health with safe, gentle, and effective remedies that even the little ones can benefit from. Learn how to incorporate castor oil into your family health regimen for lasting vitality.

Bonus 5: The Miracle Oil: Transform Your Health, Home, and Beauty Routine.
Discover the versatile wonders of castor oil in this comprehensive guide that spans health, home care, and beauty. Each tip and trick is designed to maximize the benefits of this miraculous oil, transforming the way you live.

A Call to Natural Wellness

As you turn the pages of "The Castor Oil Bible," you are not just reading another health book; you are embarking on a profound journey back to the roots of natural wellness, where every chapter serves as a stepping stone towards achieving a harmonious balance in your life. This journey is more than just an exploration—it's a reconnection with the age-old wisdom of nature and its ability to heal, nurture, and sustain us.

The pursuit of health and beauty has often been eclipsed by the rise of modern medicine and quick-fix solutions that focus more on symptoms rather than underlying causes. "The Castor Oil Bible" challenges this modern approach by reviving the traditional uses of castor oil, a remedy that has stood the test of time not only for its effectiveness but for its versatility in treating a plethora of conditions naturally.

Why settle for temporary solutions when you can opt for sustainable health? This book is not merely a collection of remedies; it's a manifesto for a life lived in closer alignment with nature's intent. Each page, each recipe, and each tip within this comprehensive guide illuminates the path to natural beauty and robust health through the potent power of castor oil.

Embark on this journey with an open heart and mind as "The Castor Oil Bible" reintroduces you to the forgotten lore of castor oil—its extraction, its rich history from ancient Egypt to its revered status in traditional healing practices across various cultures. Discover how this simple oil can be transformed into powerful serums, balms, and treatments that rejuvenate the skin, restore lustrous hair, and enhance overall wellness.

Imagine a life where your wellness routine is aligned with the rhythms of the natural world. A life where you choose holistic care over synthetic treatments. Each chapter of this book encourages this transition, offering you practical applications and methods to integrate castor oil effectively into your daily routines. Whether it's through a soothing massage oil for stress relief, a healing pack for detoxification, or a hydrating serum for timeless beauty, you'll find endless ways to harness the benefits of castor oil.

Moreover, "The Castor Oil Bible" does more than just educate—it inspires. It invites you to experiment and personalize your wellness practices, empowering you with the knowledge to create custom blends that cater to your unique health needs. This book assures you that taking control of your health is not only possible but also enjoyable.

As you delve deeper into this treasure trove of natural knowledge, let each page reaffirm your commitment to a healthier, more vibrant life. Let it remind you that the best way to honor your body is to nurture it with the healing gifts of nature. Embrace the wisdom, embrace the change, and transform how you care for your body and health.

Welcome to your new beginning. Welcome to the pure and potent world of "The Castor Oil Bible," where every drop of castor oil carries the promise of a healthier, more radiant you. Get ready to unlock the ancient secrets to health and beauty that await within these pages.

Book 1: Introduction to Castor Oil

Castor oil, a humble yet mighty oil, has journeyed through centuries, offering its rich benefits to civilizations across the globe. Extracted from the seeds of the Ricinus communis plant, this versatile oil has been a cornerstone in traditional medicine, beauty regimens, and even industrial applications. Its unique composition, primarily ricinoleic acid, sets it apart from other oils, providing a plethora of health and beauty benefits that are both profound and diverse.

The history of castor oil traces back to ancient Egypt, where it was used as a fuel in lamps, a natural remedy for ailments, and an ingredient in skincare concoctions. Its journey through time has seen it revered by various cultures for its healing properties, including in India, where it has been a staple in Ayurvedic medicine for thousands of years. The oil's ability to soothe, heal, and moisturize has made it a timeless treasure in the realm of natural health and beauty.

Understanding the science behind castor oil reveals why it is so effective. Ricinoleic acid, an unsaturated omega-9 fatty acid, is the key component that gives castor oil its remarkable anti-inflammatory, antibacterial, and antifungal properties. This makes it an excellent choice for treating skin conditions such as acne, eczema, and psoriasis, promoting hair growth, and relieving pain and inflammation.

When it comes to the types and grades of castor oil, there's a variety to choose from, each with its unique benefits. Cold-pressed castor oil retains most of its nutritional content, making it ideal for therapeutic and beauty purposes. On the other hand, Jamaican Black Castor Oil, processed differently, is renowned for its potency in promoting hair growth. Organic and hexane-free options offer purity and environmental benefits, appealing to those committed to a natural lifestyle.

Incorporating castor oil into your daily routine can be transformative. Its versatility allows it to be used in various ways, from topical applications for skin and hair care to castor oil packs for detoxification and pain relief. Whether you're looking to enhance your beauty regimen, address specific health concerns, or explore natural remedies, castor oil offers a wealth of possibilities.

As we delve deeper into the chapters (and the bonuses) that follow, we'll explore the myriad ways in which castor oil can be harnessed for health, beauty, and beyond. From DIY recipes that cater to beginners to advanced applications for specific conditions, this guide aims to empower you with the knowledge and tools to make castor oil an integral part of your wellness journey. With a focus on practical, science-backed solutions, we'll navigate the ancient and modern uses of castor oil, ensuring you can leverage its benefits to the fullest.

History and Origins of Castor Oil

The roots of castor oil's significance stretch deep into the annals of history, marking its presence in some of the earliest civilizations known to mankind. Originating from the Ricinus communis plant, the castor bean, this oil's journey through time showcases its enduring value across cultures and continents.

Ancient Egyptians were among the first to harness the benefits of castor oil, utilizing it not only as a lamp fuel but also for its potent medicinal properties. Records dating back to 4000 B.C. depict castor oil as a purgative, clearing the body of unwanted toxins. It was also a part of the beauty regimen of the Egyptian royalty, used to protect the skin and hair from the harsh desert conditions.

The castor plant, native to the Ethiopian region of East Africa, found its way to India through ancient trade routes. In India, it became a cornerstone of Ayurvedic medicine. Ayurvedic texts describe castor oil as a remedy for arthritis and digestive issues, highlighting its ability to balance Vata disorders, which are characterized by dryness and mobility. Its warming properties were believed to soothe the body's aches and stimulate digestion.

In ancient Greece, the famous physician Dioscorides noted castor oil's effectiveness in treating skin conditions, wounds, and hair growth. The Greeks, recognizing its laxative properties, named it "Kiki," a term that reflects its powerful ability to cleanse.

The spread of the castor plant continued through the Roman Empire, where it was used for lamp oil, as a natural remedy for a wide range of ailments, and even in battles, where its oil was applied to the soldiers' shields to make them slippery.

During the Middle Ages, castor oil's medicinal properties were documented in the works of Hildegard of Bingen, a renowned herbalist. She praised its use in treating skin conditions and inflammations, a testament to its enduring efficacy across centuries.

The castor oil plant was introduced to the Americas during the slave trade, where it adapted well to the tropical climate. In Jamaica, it evolved into what is now known as Jamaican Black Castor Oil, a darker, ash-rich version due to its unique processing method. This variant is highly revered for its enhanced hair growth properties.

Throughout its history, castor oil has been a versatile and powerful natural remedy. Its journey from ancient civilizations to modern times is a testament to its enduring value in natural health and beauty. As we delve deeper into the benefits and applications of castor oil, it's clear that this ancient remedy holds a special place in the holistic wellness toolkit, offering solutions for contemporary health and beauty concerns.

Ancient Uses and Cultural Significance

The reverence for castor oil in ancient civilizations was not just for its medicinal and beauty benefits but also for its profound cultural significance. This oil, derived from the humble castor bean, was more than a mere substance; it was a symbol of protection, purification, and healing that wove its way through the fabric of early societies.

In ancient Egypt, castor oil was a staple in the pharaohs' tombs, believed to aid in the journey to the afterlife. The Egyptians also used it in their lamps during religious ceremonies, casting a glow that symbolized enlightenment and guidance from the gods. This practice highlighted the oil's sacred status, transcending its everyday uses to become a part of spiritual rituals.

The cultural significance of castor oil extended to India, where it was integrated into Ayurvedic practices. Here, castor oil was not just a remedy but a holistic tool to balance the body's energies. It was used in traditional ceremonies to cleanse the body and spirit, facilitating a connection between the physical and the divine. This deep integration into spiritual practices underscores the oil's revered status in Indian culture.

In Greece, castor oil was associated with the goddess of childbirth and fertility, Hera. It was commonly used by midwives to aid in childbirth, symbolizing life and the continuation of the community. This use of castor oil in critical life moments illustrates its importance in Greek society, not just for its practical benefits but for its symbolic role in the cycle of life.

The Romans, known for their baths, incorporated castor oil into their cleansing rituals. It was used as a base for ointments and perfumes, signifying cleanliness and purity. The oil's inclusion in these rituals highlights its perceived ability to purify not just the body but the soul, making it an essential element of Roman hygiene and cosmetic practices.

In these ancient cultures, castor oil's value was multifaceted. It was a commodity, a medicinal remedy, a beauty product, and a sacred substance. Its role in religious ceremonies, health practices, and daily life illustrates a deep cultural reverence that transcended its physical properties. Castor oil was a symbol of life, purity, and connection to the divine, deeply embedded in the traditions and beliefs of early civilizations.

This rich tapestry of ancient uses and cultural significance provides a foundation for understanding how castor oil has maintained its place in modern natural health and beauty. Its ancient roots offer not just historical context but a reminder of the enduring power of natural remedies in human society.

From Ancient Egypt to Modern Times

The transition of castor oil from its ancient roots in Egypt to a staple in modern health and beauty regimens is a fascinating journey that underscores its timeless appeal and enduring benefits. As civilizations evolved, so did the applications of castor oil, expanding its reach and solidifying its place in traditional and contemporary wellness practices.

In Europe during the Renaissance, castor oil's medicinal properties were rediscovered, with herbalists and physicians prescribing it for a variety of ailments. Its use as a laxative became more widespread, and it was also applied topically to treat skin inflammations and infections. The versatility of castor oil made it a valuable commodity in the pharmacopeias of the time.

The industrial revolution brought about a new dimension to the use of castor oil. Its unique chemical structure, which makes it highly resistant to high temperatures and degradation, led to its application in the manufacturing of lubricants, hydraulic fluids, and even in early forms of plastic. This period marked the expansion of castor oil beyond medicinal and cosmetic uses, showcasing its versatility in various industrial applications.

In the 20th century, castor oil found its way into the beauty and cosmetic industry, where it was used as a key ingredient in lipsticks, shampoos, and other personal care products. Its hydrating properties made it an excellent choice for treating dry skin and hair, while its anti-inflammatory effects helped soothe irritated skin conditions.

The health food movement of the late 20th and early 21st centuries saw a resurgence in the popularity of castor oil for its natural healing properties. Health enthusiasts and holistic practitioners began to advocate for the use of castor oil packs as a detoxifying treatment, claiming benefits for liver function, immune system support, and pain relief. This period also saw a growing interest in organic and hexane-free castor oil, reflecting a broader trend towards cleaner, more sustainable health and beauty products.

Today, castor oil enjoys a revered status among natural health and beauty aficionados. Its journey from ancient Egypt to modern times is marked by a continuous discovery of its multifaceted benefits. From its early use in lamps and as a medicinal remedy to its role in industrial applications and as a key ingredient in beauty products, castor oil's versatility and efficacy have stood the test of time.

The digital age has further amplified the reach and popularity of castor oil, with countless blogs, forums, and social media platforms sharing DIY recipes and testimonials of its effectiveness. This wealth of shared knowledge has helped demystify castor oil, making it more accessible to a global audience eager to incorporate natural remedies into their health and beauty routines.

As we continue to explore the benefits and applications of castor oil, it's clear that this ancient oil has seamlessly integrated into the fabric of modern wellness practices. Its enduring legacy is a testament to the power of natural remedies and the timeless pursuit of health and beauty.

Traditional Healing Practices Across Cultures

Across the globe, traditional healing practices have long embraced castor oil for its remarkable therapeutic properties. From the Americas to Asia, each culture has discovered and harnessed the oil's benefits in unique and profound ways, integrating it into their healing traditions and daily wellness routines.

In the Caribbean, particularly in Jamaica, castor oil has been a staple in folk medicine for generations. Known locally as "black castor oil," its preparation involves roasting the beans before pressing, a method believed to increase its potency. Jamaicans have traditionally used this oil to treat a wide range of conditions, from muscle aches and arthritis to skin conditions and hair growth. The oil's deep penetration is thought to stimulate circulation, promote healing, and restore balance within the body.

Moving to the East, in India, castor oil's integration into Ayurvedic medicine showcases its versatility and esteemed status among natural remedies. Ayurveda, which emphasizes balance in bodily systems, uses castor oil to harmonize the doshas (body energies) and cleanse the body of ama (toxins). It is commonly used in Panchakarma, a detoxification process, where castor oil is ingested to induce purgation, effectively cleansing the digestive system. Additionally, its anti-inflammatory properties make it a go-to treatment for joint pain and swelling, aligning with Ayurveda's holistic approach to health and wellness.

In Africa, particularly within Ethiopian traditional medicine, castor oil has been used to treat skin infections and as a natural moisturizer to protect the skin in harsh climates. Its antibacterial and antifungal properties are valued for wound healing, demonstrating the oil's broad-spectrum utility in various African healing practices.

In traditional Chinese medicine (TCM), castor oil is used externally, often in the form of poultices or compresses. TCM practitioners apply it to areas of stagnation or discomfort, where its warming and invigorating qualities help to unblock Qi (vital energy) and promote healing. This external application aligns with TCM's emphasis on external treatments for internal conditions, showcasing castor oil's adaptability to different therapeutic philosophies.

In the Mediterranean region, particularly in traditional Greek medicine, castor oil was known as a powerful laxative and was also applied topically to treat skin irritations and infections. Its use in ancient Greece laid the groundwork for its later adoption in European folk medicine, where it was used to treat a variety of ailments, from gastrointestinal issues to inflammatory conditions.

These diverse practices across cultures not only highlight the universal appeal of castor oil but also demonstrate the shared human instinct to turn to nature for healing. Despite the vast geographical and cultural distances, the traditional use of castor oil as a healing agent forms a common thread, weaving together the wisdom of generations and the innate human connection to the natural world.

As we explore the multifaceted uses of castor oil in traditional healing practices, it becomes clear that this ancient remedy holds a special place in the heart of natural medicine worldwide. Its enduring presence in cultural healing traditions speaks to its effectiveness and the deep-rooted belief in its power to heal, soothe, and rejuvenate the body and spirit.

The Science Behind Castor Oil

Ricinoleic acid, the powerhouse behind castor oil's myriad of benefits, distinguishes this natural remedy from others in your wellness toolkit. This unique fatty acid is responsible for most of castor oil's therapeutic properties, including its anti-inflammatory, antibacterial, and antifungal effects. Understanding how ricinoleic acid works at the molecular level can help demystify the science behind why castor oil is such a versatile and effective natural treatment for a wide range of conditions.

Firstly, ricinoleic acid acts as a powerful anti-inflammatory agent. When applied topically, it penetrates the skin and inhibits the production of substances that cause inflammation. This makes castor oil an excellent choice for conditions like acne, eczema, and psoriasis, where inflammation plays a key role. The mechanism involves the ricinoleic acid binding to specific receptors on the cells of the skin, which then modulate the immune response, reducing swelling and redness.

Moreover, castor oil's antibacterial properties are largely attributed to ricinoleic acid's ability to disrupt the cell membranes of bacteria. This disruption inhibits the bacteria's ability to grow and reproduce, effectively stopping infections in their tracks. This action is particularly beneficial for treating minor cuts, abrasions, and skin infections, providing a natural, chemical-free method to keep wounds clean and promote healing.

The antifungal effects of castor oil, again, are credited to ricinoleic acid. It works by penetrating the fungal cell wall and inducing cell death, making it an effective treatment for conditions like athlete's foot, ringworm, and scalp infections caused by fungi. Unlike many antifungal treatments that can be harsh on the skin, castor oil provides a gentler alternative that can soothe the skin while actively fighting fungal infections.

In addition to these properties, ricinoleic acid is also known to be effective in promoting circulation. When applied in the form of a castor oil pack, it can enhance blood flow to the area, which is beneficial for healing and detoxification processes. This increased circulation can help in the removal of toxins from the tissue, thereby relieving pain and inflammation not only on the surface but deep within the body as well.

Furthermore, castor oil's hydrating properties stem from its ability to lock moisture into the skin. Ricinoleic acid, being a humectant, attracts water to the skin, keeping it hydrated and plump. This is particularly beneficial for dry skin conditions and for maintaining healthy, hydrated skin and hair. The oil forms a barrier that prevents water loss, ensuring that the skin remains supple and hair retains its moisture, enhancing elasticity and preventing breakage.

Lastly, the role of castor oil in promoting hair growth and scalp health can be linked to ricinoleic acid's ability to balance the pH of the scalp, cleanse toxins that impede hair growth, and provide essential nutrients to hair follicles. This multifaceted approach not only supports hair growth but also improves the health of the scalp, leading to thicker, stronger, and more lustrous hair.

In summary, the science behind castor oil's effectiveness is deeply rooted in the properties of ricinoleic acid. This unique compound provides a natural, holistic way to address a variety of health and beauty concerns, from skin and hair care to anti-inflammatory and pain relief applications. By harnessing the power of ricinoleic acid, castor oil offers a safe, effective, and versatile solution for those seeking natural remedies.

Key Components: Ricinoleic Acid and Omega-9 Fatty Acids

Ricinoleic acid and omega-9 fatty acids stand at the heart of castor oil's remarkable health and beauty benefits. Ricinoleic acid, a monounsaturated fatty acid unique to castor oil, comprises about 90% of its fatty acid content, making it a potent ingredient in natural remedies. Its structure allows it to deeply penetrate the skin and scalp, delivering powerful anti-inflammatory, antibacterial, and antifungal effects. This makes it an invaluable ally against acne, dandruff, and various skin conditions, promoting healing from within.

Omega-9 fatty acids, also present in castor oil, are known for their moisturizing and regenerative properties. They play a crucial role in stimulating healthy hair growth, enhancing skin health, and supporting the body's natural inflammatory response. Unlike other fatty acids, the body cannot produce omega-9s in significant amounts, making external sources like castor oil essential for maintaining optimal health.

- Anti-inflammatory Benefits: Ricinoleic acid's anti-inflammatory properties make castor oil a natural treatment for swollen joints, muscle aches, and even arthritis. By applying castor oil directly to the affected area, you can reduce inflammation and alleviate pain without the need for synthetic medications.

- Antibacterial and Antifungal Properties: The unique composition of castor oil allows it to fight off bacterial and fungal infections, promoting a healthy scalp and skin. It's particularly effective in treating fungal conditions like athlete's foot, ringworm, and scalp infections, offering a natural alternative to harsh chemical treatments.

- Moisturizing and Healing: Omega-9 fatty acids in castor oil help lock in moisture, keeping the skin hydrated and plump. This not only prevents dryness but also helps reduce the appearance of wrinkles and fine lines, promoting a youthful, radiant complexion.

- Promoting Hair Growth: The combination of ricinoleic acid and omega-9 fatty acids makes castor oil a powerful stimulant for hair growth. By improving circulation to the scalp and providing essential nutrients to hair follicles, it can help reverse hair loss and encourage the growth of thicker, healthier hair.

Incorporating castor oil into your beauty and wellness routine can thus offer a multitude of benefits, thanks to these key components. Whether used topically or as part of a castor oil pack, its natural healing properties can support your body's health in a holistic, gentle manner.

How Castor Oil Benefits Skin, Hair, and Overall Health

Castor oil, a treasure trove of ricinoleic acid and omega-9 fatty acids, offers a myriad of benefits for skin, hair, and overall health that are both impressive and wide-ranging. Its unique composition allows it to penetrate deeply into the skin and scalp, delivering nourishment, hydration, and healing properties from the inside out. Here's how castor oil can be a game-changer in your health and beauty regimen:

- Skin Health: Castor oil is a natural emollient, providing much-needed moisture to dry, irritated skin. By creating a protective barrier on the skin's surface, it prevents water loss, keeping the skin hydrated and plump. This hydration is key in maintaining a youthful appearance, as well-cared-for skin appears smoother and less prone to the development of fine lines and wrinkles. For those battling acne, the antibacterial properties of castor oil can help fight off bacteria that contribute to breakouts, while its anti-inflammatory effects reduce redness and swelling.

- Hair Care: The benefits of castor oil extend to hair health by nourishing the scalp and strengthening the roots. Its ricinoleic acid content helps balance scalp pH, rejuvenating the scalp and promoting healthier hair growth. By improving blood circulation to the scalp, castor oil ensures that hair follicles receive the nutrients they need to produce stronger, thicker hair. Additionally, its moisture-sealing properties help combat dryness and brittleness, making hair shinier and more resilient against breakage.

- Anti-inflammatory Properties: Beyond beauty, castor oil's anti-inflammatory capabilities make it a valuable ally against joint pain and inflammation. Applying castor oil directly to sore areas can alleviate discomfort, making it a simple yet effective remedy for those with arthritis or muscle pain. Its ability to penetrate deeply means it can help reduce inflammation not just on the surface, but also within the underlying tissues.

- Immune System Support: The use of castor oil packs, a popular application method, has been shown to support lymphatic drainage and improve immune function. By enhancing the body's ability to detoxify and fight off infections, castor oil can contribute to overall health and well-being. This detoxifying effect is also beneficial for digestive health, as it can help relieve constipation and promote regular bowel movements.

- Antimicrobial Effects: Castor oil's antimicrobial properties make it a potent remedy for fungal and bacterial skin infections. Whether it's athlete's foot, ringworm, or scalp infections, applying castor oil to the affected area can help eradicate the infection, thanks to its ability to penetrate the skin and act directly on the pathogens.

Incorporating castor oil into your daily routine can thus offer comprehensive benefits, addressing everything from skin and hair care needs to supporting your body's natural healing processes. Whether applied topically, used in hair treatments, or as part of a castor oil pack, its versatility and efficacy make castor oil a must-have in your natural health arsenal.

Research Studies Supporting Castor Oil's Benefits

The efficacy of castor oil in various health and beauty applications is not just anecdotal; it is backed by scientific research that underscores its benefits. Studies have delved into the properties of ricinoleic acid, a major component of castor oil, revealing its potential in anti-inflammatory, antimicrobial, and healing capacities.

One significant study published in the International Journal of Toxicology assessed the safety of castor oil as a cosmetic ingredient, concluding that it is safe for use in cosmetic formulations. This study is crucial for those concerned about the safety of natural products, providing peace of mind that castor oil is a safe addition to beauty routines.

Research in the Journal of Ethnopharmacology explored the analgesic and anti-inflammatory effects of ricinoleic acid, finding that it effectively reduces pain and swelling when applied topically. This supports the traditional use of castor oil packs for relieving joint pain, arthritis, and muscle aches, offering a natural alternative to over-the-counter pain relievers.

Another study focused on the antimicrobial properties of castor oil, demonstrating its effectiveness against bacterial strains such as Staphylococcus aureus and Escherichia coli. This research validates the use of castor oil in treating minor cuts, wounds, and skin infections, highlighting its role as a natural antiseptic.

The role of castor oil in promoting hair growth has also been the subject of scientific inquiry. A study in the Journal of Cosmetic Science reported that castor oil could increase the luster of hair, suggesting that its application contributes to healthier, shinier hair. While direct evidence of castor oil stimulating hair growth is limited, its nourishing properties support scalp health, which is essential for healthy hair growth.

Furthermore, castor oil's hydrating effects on the skin have been documented in dermatological research. Its ability to retain moisture and enhance skin barrier function makes it an effective treatment for dry skin conditions, eczema, and psoriasis. By maintaining skin hydration, castor oil helps to keep the skin looking youthful and radiant.

In the realm of digestive health, the laxative properties of castor oil have been well-documented. A study published in Alternative Therapies in Health and Medicine examined its use in constipation, confirming that castor oil acts as a stimulant laxative, providing relief for those suffering from constipation.

These studies, among others, provide a scientific foundation for the benefits of castor oil, bridging traditional knowledge with modern research. By understanding the research-backed advantages of castor oil, individuals can confidently incorporate this natural remedy into their health and beauty practices, leveraging its myriad benefits for improved well-being and natural beauty.

Types and Grades of Castor Oil

Understanding the different types and grades of castor oil is crucial for maximizing its benefits for your health and beauty routines. Each type has unique properties and uses, making it important to choose the right one for your specific needs.

- Cold-Pressed Castor Oil: This type is always extracted directly from the castor bean without using heat. The cold-pressing process helps retain most of the oil's nutritional content, making it rich in vitamins and minerals. Cold-pressed castor oil is considered the highest quality for cosmetic and medicinal purposes due to its purity and high concentration of ricinoleic acid. It's ideal for skin and hair treatments, offering deep hydration and promoting growth.

- Refined Castor Oil: Refined castor oil undergoes a heating process and sometimes chemical treatment to remove impurities and reduce its odor and color. While it's still effective for industrial and some cosmetic applications, it may lack some of the nutritional benefits of cold-pressed oil. This type is commonly used in manufacturing, particularly in the production of soaps, lubricants, and other products.

- Organic Castor Oil: Certified organic castor oil is extracted from castor beans grown without the use of pesticides, fertilizers, or genetically modified organisms (GMOs). For those committed to an organic lifestyle, this type ensures that you're using a product free from synthetic additives. Organic castor oil is often cold-pressed, preserving its health benefits and making it suitable for all beauty and health applications.

- Hexane-Free Castor Oil: Some castor oils are extracted using hexane, a solvent that can help increase the yield of oil from each bean. However, hexane-free castor oil is preferred by health-conscious consumers. The absence of hexane in the extraction process ensures that the oil remains free from chemical residues, making it safer for use on skin and hair.

- Jamaican Black Castor Oil: This variety is processed differently from other types. The beans are first roasted, then ground into a paste before being boiled to extract the oil. The result is a dark-colored oil with an ash content that is believed to provide additional benefits for hair growth. Jamaican Black Castor Oil is highly revered for its ability to strengthen, thicken, and promote healthy hair growth. It's also used for a variety of scalp issues, such as dandruff and dry scalp.

- Deodorized Castor Oil: For those who prefer a less noticeable scent, deodorized castor oil undergoes a treatment to reduce its natural, nutty aroma. While it retains most of the oil's beneficial properties, the deodorization process can make it more appealing for use in homemade skincare and haircare formulations where a neutral scent is desired.

Choosing the right type of castor oil depends on your specific needs and preferences. For most health and beauty applications, cold-pressed, organic, or Jamaican Black Castor Oil are the best choices due to their high quality and nutrient content. Whether you're looking to improve your skin and hair health, relieve pain and inflammation, or explore natural remedies, understanding these types and grades of castor oil will help you make informed decisions and achieve the best results.

Cold-Pressed vs. Refined Castor Oil

When exploring the world of castor oil, understanding the distinction between cold-pressed and refined varieties is crucial for harnessing its full potential in your health and beauty regimen. Each type offers unique benefits and applications, making it essential to choose the right one for your specific needs.

Cold-pressed castor oil is extracted from the castor beans without the application of heat, ensuring that the oil retains its natural healing properties and nutritional content. This method preserves the integrity of essential fatty acids, vitamins, and minerals, making cold-pressed castor oil highly prized for its therapeutic and cosmetic applications. Its rich concentration of ricinoleic acid, a potent anti-inflammatory and antibacterial agent, makes it an excellent choice for skin and hair treatments. Cold-pressed castor oil is ideal for those looking to leverage castor oil's natural benefits without compromising on quality. It is particularly effective in:

- Moisturizing and nourishing the skin, helping to restore elasticity and reduce signs of aging.

- Promoting hair growth by improving scalp health and strengthening hair roots.

- Soothing inflamed skin conditions such as eczema, psoriasis, and acne due to its anti-inflammatory properties.

Refined castor oil, on the other hand, undergoes a heating process and may be treated with chemicals to remove impurities, deodorize, and bleach the oil. This results in a product that is odorless and colorless, with a more neutral profile suitable for various industrial and cosmetic applications. While refined castor oil still offers benefits such as moisturizing properties and the ability to soothe irritated skin, the refining process can diminish its nutritional content and therapeutic potency. Refined castor oil is commonly used in:

- Manufacturing processes, including the production of soaps, lubricants, and other industrial products.

- Cosmetic formulations where the absence of scent and color is preferred, making it a versatile carrier oil for beauty products.

Choosing between cold-pressed and refined castor oil depends largely on your intended use. For therapeutic and beauty purposes, cold-pressed castor oil is the superior choice due to its higher quality and concentration of beneficial compounds. Its ability to deeply nourish and heal makes it a staple in natural health and beauty routines. However, if you're formulating products where the scent and color of castor oil might be an issue, or if the oil is intended for industrial use, refined castor oil could be the more appropriate option.

Incorporating the right type of castor oil into your regimen can significantly enhance your health and beauty practices, offering a natural, effective solution to a wide range of concerns. Whether you opt for the holistic benefits of cold-pressed castor oil or the versatility of refined castor oil, understanding these differences ensures you can make informed decisions that align with your wellness and cosmetic goals.

Organic and Hexane-Free Castor Oil

Organic and Hexane-Free Castor Oil

Choosing organic and hexane-free castor oil is a pivotal step for those committed to a holistic and environmentally conscious lifestyle. This type of castor oil ensures that the product is not only free from harmful chemical residues but also produced in a way that supports sustainable farming practices. Here's a deeper look into why organic and hexane-free castor oil stands out and how it can be integrated into your wellness and beauty routines.

Organic castor oil is extracted from castor beans grown without the use of synthetic pesticides, fertilizers, or genetically modified organisms (GMOs). This approach not only preserves the purity of the oil but also contributes to the health of the soil and the surrounding ecosystem. When you opt for organic castor oil, you're choosing a product that supports the planet's well-being alongside your own.

Hexane-free castor oil takes this commitment a step further by ensuring that the extraction process is free from hexane, a petroleum-based solvent. While hexane is often used in the oil extraction process to increase yield, it can leave behind trace amounts of chemical residue. Hexane-free castor oil is extracted using mechanical methods or alternative solvents that pose no risk to your health, making it the safer choice for topical and internal use.

Here are some benefits and uses of organic and hexane-free castor oil:

- Skin Care: Its purity makes it ideal for sensitive skin types. Use it as a moisturizer to hydrate and replenish the skin, or apply it to areas of inflammation for its soothing effects.

- Hair Health: Rich in nutrients and free from contaminants, this oil can help promote a healthy scalp and stronger hair growth. Massage it into your scalp to balance oil production and stimulate hair follicles.

- Health Remedies: Organic and hexane-free castor oil is safe for making castor oil packs, a popular treatment for detoxification and pain relief. Its clean profile ensures that you're not introducing toxins to your body during the process.

- Environmental Impact: By choosing organic and hexane-free products, you're supporting farming practices that minimize soil depletion and pollution, contributing to a healthier planet.

Incorporating organic and hexane-free castor oil into your routine is straightforward. For skin applications, start with a small amount, as a little goes a long way. For hair treatments, warm the oil slightly for deeper penetration and cover with a shower cap for an intensive overnight treatment. When making castor oil packs, ensure the cloth is saturated but not dripping, and always use a heat source to activate its therapeutic properties.

In essence, opting for organic and hexane-free castor oil is a choice that benefits not only your personal health and beauty but also the environment. Its superior quality and safety profile make it a valuable addition to any natural wellness regimen, offering peace of mind that you're using a product that is as clean and green as it is effective.

Black Castor Oil vs. Regular Castor Oil

Black Castor Oil vs. Regular Castor Oil

When exploring the world of castor oil for health and beauty, you'll likely come across two main types: Black Castor Oil and Regular Castor Oil. Both have their unique benefits and uses, making them valuable additions to your natural wellness and beauty routines. Understanding the differences between these two can help you make an informed decision on which is best suited for your specific needs.

Black Castor Oil, often referred to as Jamaican Black Castor Oil (JBCO), is processed differently than regular castor oil. The beans are first roasted, then ground into a paste before being boiled to extract the oil. This method results in a dark color and a burnt, smoky scent. The ash content, a result of the roasting process, is believed to contribute to its enhanced benefits, particularly for hair growth. JBCO is renowned for its ability to strengthen, thicken, and promote healthy hair growth. It's also used for a variety of scalp issues, such as dandruff and dry scalp. The high ash content is thought to increase its potency, making it a favorite for those looking to boost hair health.

Regular Castor Oil, on the other hand, is typically cold-pressed from the castor beans without roasting, resulting in a pale yellow color and a milder scent. This type retains most of the natural nutrients found in castor beans, including ricinoleic acid, which is known for its anti-inflammatory, antibacterial, and moisturizing properties. Regular castor oil is incredibly versatile, used not only for hair care but also for skin hydration, reducing inflammation, and even as a laxative. Its lighter texture and composition make it suitable for a wide range of cosmetic and medicinal applications.

Here are some considerations to help you decide between Black Castor Oil and Regular Castor Oil:

- Hair Care: If your primary goal is to improve hair health, Jamaican Black Castor Oil might be your best choice due to its reputation for promoting hair growth and strengthening hair. Its rich nutrients and ash content are particularly beneficial for those with dry, brittle, or damaged hair.

- Skin Care: For general skin care purposes, including moisturizing dry skin, treating acne, or reducing the appearance of scars, Regular Castor Oil is highly effective. Its lighter consistency makes it easier to apply and absorb into the skin without leaving a heavy residue.

- Purity and Processing: If you prefer minimally processed products, cold-pressed Regular Castor

Oil maintains a closer composition to the natural state of the castor bean. It undergoes less processing, which may appeal to purists or those with sensitive skin.

- Texture and Scent: Consider your preference for texture and scent. Jamaican Black Castor Oil has a thicker consistency and a smoky smell, which some may find overpowering. Regular Castor Oil is lighter and has a much milder scent, making it more versatile for blending with other ingredients in DIY beauty recipes.

Incorporating either Black Castor Oil or Regular Castor Oil into your routine can offer significant health and beauty benefits. Whether you're looking to enhance your hair care regimen, improve your skin health, or seek a natural remedy for inflammation, choosing the right type of castor oil can help you achieve your wellness goals.

Book 2: Preparing and Using Castor Oil

Safe Preparation and Application

Ensuring the safe preparation and application of castor oil is paramount to harnessing its full benefits without any adverse effects. Here are some guidelines to follow:

1. Choose the Right Type of Castor Oil: Opt for cold-pressed, organic, or Jamaican Black Castor Oil for beauty and health applications. These types retain the most nutrients and are free from harmful processing chemicals.

2. Patch Test: Before applying castor oil to a larger area of your skin or scalp, do a patch test. Apply a small amount on your inner arm and wait for at least 24 hours to check for any allergic reaction or irritation.

3. Cleanse the Area: Whether you're applying castor oil to your skin, scalp, or as part of a castor oil pack, always start with a clean surface. Gently cleanse the area with a mild cleanser and pat dry.

4. Warm the Oil: Slightly warming the oil can enhance its penetration and effectiveness. Warm the oil by placing the bottle in a bowl of hot water for a few minutes. Test the oil on one of your wrist to ensure it's warm but not hot.

5. Apply Sparingly: A little goes a long way with castor oil due to its thick consistency. Start with a small amount, and gently massage it into the skin, scalp, or hair. For hair and scalp treatments, you can use a dropper for better control and distribution.

6. Use a Protective Barrier: If using castor oil overnight, especially in hair treatments or castor oil packs, protect your linens and clothing. Cover the treated area with a plastic cap or wrap, and place an old towel on your pillow.

7. Rinse Thoroughly: After application, especially with hair treatments, ensure you rinse the oil out thoroughly with a gentle shampoo. It may require two washes to remove all oil residues.

8. Frequency of Use: For skin treatments, using castor oil 2-3 times a week is sufficient. For hair growth treatments, applying it once a week can yield good results. Listen to your body's response and adjust accordingly.

Dos and Don'ts of Applying Castor Oil

- Do use castor oil as part of your nighttime routine to allow ample time for absorption.
- Don't use castor oil on broken skin or open wounds without consulting a healthcare provider.
- Do combine castor oil with lighter carrier oils like almond or coconut oil for easier application

and absorption, especially for hair and scalp treatments.

- Don't ingest castor oil without the guidance of a healthcare professional, as it can act as a potent laxative.
- Do store castor oil in a cool, dark place to preserve its shelf life and effectiveness.

How to Make Castor Oil Packs for Detox and Healing

Castor oil packs are a traditional remedy for detoxification, pain relief, and supporting digestive health. Here's how to make and use them:

Materials Needed:

- High-quality, cold-pressed castor oil

- A piece of wool flannel or cotton cloth

- Plastic wrap (optional, to prevent staining)

- A hot water bottle or heating pad

- An old towel or sheet

Step-by-Step Instructions:

1. Prepare the Cloth: Cut the cloth to a size large enough to cover the targeted area, such as the abdomen for digestive issues or a joint for pain relief.
2. Saturate the Cloth: Soak the cloth in castor oil until it is fully saturated but not dripping.

3. Apply to the Targeted Area: Place the saturated cloth on the targeted area. Cover it with plastic wrap if desired, to prevent oil stains.

4. Add Heat: Place a hot water bottle or heating pad over the pack to help the oil penetrate deeper into the skin. The heat also aids in relaxation and increases the effectiveness of the treatment.

5. Rest: Lie down and relax with the pack in place for 45-60 minutes. This is an excellent time for meditation or deep breathing exercises.

6. Clean Up: Remove the pack then clean the area with a diluted water solution and baking soda to remove any oil residue. Store the cloth in a plastic bag in the refrigerator. It can be reused up to 30 times.

Safety Tips:

- Ensure the heat source is not too hot to prevent burns.

- Avoid using castor oil packs during pregnancy or menstruation without consulting a healthcare provider.

- If you have a medical condition, consult a healthcare professional before using castor oil packs.

Storage and Shelf Life: Keeping Your Castor Oil Fresh

- Store castor oil in a cool, dark place to maintain its potency.

- Tightly seal the bottle after each use to prevent oxidation.

- Quality castor oil can last up to a year if stored properly. If it smells rancid or unusual, it's time to replace it.

By following these guidelines, you can safely prepare and use castor oil to tap into its ancient healing properties for modern wellness benefits.

Safe Preparation and Application

Choosing the right type of castor oil is the first crucial step in ensuring its safe and effective use. For health and beauty applications, prioritize cold-pressed, organic, or Jamaican Black Castor Oil. These varieties maintain the integrity of the oil's beneficial properties without the addition of harmful chemicals.

Before incorporating castor oil into your routine, conducting a patch test is essential to avoid potential allergic reactions. Apply a small amount of oil to a discreet area of your skin, such as the inner wrist or elbow, and wait for at least 24 hours to observe any signs of irritation or discomfort. If any adverse reactions occur, discontinue use immediately and consult a healthcare provider.

When preparing to apply castor oil, especially to the skin or scalp, cleanliness cannot be overstated. Begin with a clean surface by gently washing the area with a mild cleanser, ensuring that you are working with a fresh canvas to maximize the oil's benefits.

Warming the oil slightly can enhance its therapeutic effects, making it more penetrable and soothing upon application. Warm the oil by placing the bottle in a bowl of hot water for a few minutes, ensuring it reaches a comfortable temperature that will not cause discomfort or burns upon application.

In application, moderation is key. Castor oil is notably thick and can go a long way with just a small quantity. Start with a modest amount, gently massaging it into the skin, scalp, or hair, depending on your treatment area. For hair and scalp treatments, consider using a dropper for more precise control and even distribution.

Protecting your linens and clothing is advisable when using castor oil, especially in overnight treatments. Cover the treated area with a suitable wrap or wear old clothes that you don't mind getting oily. For hair treatments, a shower cap or towel can prevent oil transfer to pillows and bedding.

Rinsing castor oil out, particularly from hair, requires thoroughness. Due to its viscosity, you may need to shampoo twice to fully remove the oil, ensuring no residue is left that could weigh down your hair or attract dirt.

The frequency of castor oil application will vary depending on its purpose. For skin treatments, two to three times a week is generally sufficient. For promoting hair growth, a weekly application can offer significant benefits. Pay attention to how your body responds and adjust the frequency accordingly to suit your individual needs.

In summary, the safe preparation and application of castor oil involve selecting the appropriate type, performing a patch test, starting with a clean area, warming the oil, applying sparingly, protecting surfaces from oil stains, thoroughly rinsing after use, and adjusting frequency as needed. By following these guidelines, you can enjoy the myriad benefits of castor oil while minimizing any risks of adverse reactions or inconvenience.

Dos and Don'ts of Applying Castor Oil

Do:

- Test for Allergies: Always perform a patch test before using castor oil extensively. Apply a small amount on your inner wrist and wait for 24 hours. If there's no adverse reaction, you're likely safe to proceed.

- Use the Right Type: For beauty and health applications, opt for cold-pressed, organic castor oil. Its purity and nutrient content are superior.

- Warm It Up: Gently warming castor oil can enhance its effectiveness, especially for hair and skin treatments. Warm oil helps in better penetration and soothing action.

- Mix with Carrier Oils: If you find castor oil too thick or sticky, dilute it with a lighter carrier oil like almond, coconut, or jojoba oil. This makes it easier to apply and spread.

- Apply with Care: Use a cotton ball or your fingertips to apply castor oil. For hair treatments, a dropper can help in applying the oil directly to the scalp.

- Protect Your Linens: Castor oil can stain, so cover your pillow with an old towel or use a shower cap when leaving it on overnight.

Don't:

- Overapply: A little goes a long way. Using too much castor oil can lead to greasiness and may clog pores, especially on the face.

- Ignore Reactions: If you experience any irritation, redness, or discomfort after applying castor oil, stop using it immediately and wash the area with water.

- Use on Broken Skin: Avoid applying castor oil on cuts, open wounds, or broken skin unless advised by a healthcare professional.

- Forget to Wash Off: For certain applications, especially on the face or hair, ensure you thoroughly wash off the castor oil to prevent buildup or irritation.

- Neglect Storage Instructions: Keep your castor oil in a cool, dark place to maintain its efficacy. Improper storage can lead to rancidity or loss of beneficial properties.

- Apply Near Eyes Without Caution: Be extremely careful if using castor oil near the eyes, such as for eyelash growth. Avoid direct contact with the eyes to prevent irritation.

By adhering to these dos and don'ts, you can safely and effectively incorporate castor oil into your beauty and wellness routines, leveraging its numerous benefits without unwanted side effects.

How to Make Castor Oil Packs for Detox and Healing

Materials Needed:

- High-quality, cold-pressed castor oil

- Cotton or wool flannel large enough to cover the affected area

- Plastic wrap or a large plastic bag

- A hot water bottle or heating pad

- An old towel or sheet to protect bedding or clothing

- Safety pins or clips (optional, to secure the pack in place)

Step-by-Step Instructions:

1. Begin by folding the flannel or cotton cloth into layers, ensuring it's large enough to cover the targeted area but not so large that it becomes unwieldy. The cloth should be thick enough to hold a generous amount of castor oil but not so saturated that it drips excessively.

2. Pour castor oil over the cloth slowly, allowing it to soak in evenly. The goal is for the cloth to be well-saturated but not dripping wet. You can do this in a large bowl or directly over the sink to avoid messes. Depending on the size of your cloth, you may need a quarter to a half cup of castor oil.

3. Once the cloth is saturated, if you haven't already, lie down on an old towel or sheet that you don't mind getting oily. Place the saturated cloth directly on your skin over the area you wish to target, such as the abdomen for detoxification or a joint for pain relief.

4. Cover the saturated cloth with plastic wrap or place it inside a large plastic bag. This layer is to prevent the oil from staining your heating pad or hot water bottle and to keep the heat in.

5. Place a hot water bottle or a heating pad over the plastic-covered cloth. The heat will help the castor oil penetrate more deeply into the skin and underlying tissues, enhancing its therapeutic effects. Ensure the heat is comfortable and not too hot to avoid burns.

6. Relax with the castor oil pack in place for about 45-60 minutes. This is an excellent time to practice deep breathing, meditate, or simply rest. The combination of castor oil and heat can aid in relaxation and promote healing.

7. After the time is up, remove the pack and cleanse the area with a warm, damp washcloth. You might find that a mixture of baking soda and water helps remove any residual oil more effectively.

8. Store the used castor oil pack in a plastic bag in the refrigerator. You can reuse the pack multiple times, adding more oil as needed to keep it saturated. It's generally recommended to replace the pack after it starts to change color or smell, typically after 30 uses.

Safety Tips:

- Always check the temperature of your heat source before applying it to your skin to prevent burns.

- Castor oil packs are generally safe for most people, but it's wise to consult with a healthcare provider before using them, especially if you are pregnant, nursing, or have any medical conditions.

- Avoid using castor oil packs if you have open wounds, rashes, or infections in the area you're treating.

By incorporating castor oil packs into your wellness routine, you can harness the detoxifying and healing properties of castor oil, promoting relaxation, pain relief, and overall well-being.

Storage and Shelf Life: Keeping Your Castor Oil Fresh

To ensure your castor oil retains its therapeutic properties and remains safe for use, proper storage is essential. Castor oil, like many natural oils, can degrade over time when exposed to air, light, and heat. Here are practical steps to maximize the shelf life of your castor oil and keep it fresh for as long as possible:

- Cool and Dark Storage: Store your castor oil in a cool, dark place away from direct sunlight. A cupboard away from heat sources like stoves or heaters is ideal. Be aware that exposure to some light or heat might accelerate the oxidation and lead to rancidity.

- Airtight Containers: Keep castor oil in an airtight container to minimize its exposure to air. Oxygen can react with the oil, causing it to spoil more quickly. If your castor oil didn't come in a dark, glass bottle, consider transferring it to one. Dark glass bottles help block light and prevent oxidation.

- Refrigeration for Longevity: For long-term storage, consider refrigerating your castor oil. Lower temperatures slow down the degradation process, extending the oil's shelf life. However, castor oil may thicken or become cloudy when refrigerated, which is normal. Simply allow the oil to come to room temperature before use, and it will return to its original consistency.

- Label and Date: Mark the purchase date on the bottle. Even with optimal storage conditions, castor oil should ideally be used within a year of opening. Keeping track of when you opened the oil can help you use it when it's most potent.

- Check for Signs of Spoilage: Periodically check your castor oil for signs of spoilage, including changes in color, consistency, or smell. Fresh castor oil should have a light, pale yellow color and a mild, characteristic scent.

- Proper Handling: Each time you use your castor oil, make sure your hands and any utensils you use are clean to avoid contaminating the oil with bacteria or other substances that could promote spoilage.

- Small Batches: If you use castor oil infrequently, consider purchasing smaller bottles to ensure you can use it up before it begins to degrade. This approach minimizes waste and ensures the oil is fresh when you use it.

By following these storage tips, you can preserve the quality and efficacy of your castor oil, ensuring it remains a valuable addition to your health and beauty routine. Properly stored castor oil will maintain its beneficial properties, allowing you to enjoy its full range of uses without concern for degradation or spoilage.

DIY Castor Oil Recipes for Beginners

Unlock the natural power of castor oil with these simple, effective DIY recipes tailored for beginners.

Whether you're looking to enhance your beauty routine or find natural solutions for common health concerns, these recipes are designed to be easy to follow, using ingredients that are readily accessible.

1. Nourishing Hair Mask for Growth and Shine

Materials:
- 2 tablespoons of cold-pressed castor oil
- 1 tablespoon of coconut oil
- A few drops of rosemary essential oil (optional for added benefits)

Instructions:

1. In a small bowl, mix the castor oil and coconut oil. If your coconut oil is solid, gently warm it to liquid form.

2. Add a few drops of rosemary essential oil to the mixture. Rosemary oil can stimulate hair growth and add a pleasant scent.

3. Apply the mixture to your scalp and hair, massaging gently for a few minutes to ensure even distribution and to stimulate the scalp.

4. Cover your hair with a shower cap and leave the mask on for at least an hour, or overnight for deeper conditioning.

5. Wash your hair thoroughly with a gentle shampoo to remove the oil. You may need to shampoo twice to get rid of the oiliness.

6. Gentle Castor Oil Face Cleanser for Glowing Skin

Materials:
- 1 tablespoon of castor oil
- 2 tablespoons of sweet almond oil or olive oil

Instructions:

1. Combine the castor oil with your choice of sweet almond oil or olive oil in a small bottle. Shake well to mix.

2. Pour a small amount of the oil blend into your palms and gently massage onto your dry face. The oil will help lift any dirt and makeup from your skin.

3. Soak a clean washcloth in hot water, wring out the excess, and place it over your face. The steam will help open your pores and allow the oils to penetrate deeply.

4. Once the washcloth cools, use it to gently wipe away the oil. Rinse your face with cool water to close the pores.

5. Pat your face dry with a clean towel. Your skin should feel clean, moisturized, and soft.

6. Soothing Castor Oil Pack for Digestive Comfort

Materials:
- High-quality, cold-pressed castor oil
- A piece of wool flannel or cotton cloth
- Plastic wrap
- A hot water bottle or heating pad
- An old towel

Instructions:

1. Fold the cloth to a size that covers the targeted area, such as your abdomen.

2. Saturate the cloth with castor oil, ensuring it's fully soaked but not dripping.

3. Place the cloth on your abdomen and cover it with plastic wrap to avoid staining your clothes or bedding.

4. Lay the hot water bottle or heating pad over the plastic wrap to add warmth, which enhances the oil's penetration and effectiveness.

5. Relax and let the pack sit for 45-60 minutes. Use this time to rest or meditate.

6. Remove the pack and cleanse the area with a warm, damp cloth. You can store the cloth in a plastic bag in the fridge for future use.

7. Castor Oil Eyelash and Eyebrow Serum for Fuller Look

Materials:
- 1 teaspoon of castor oil
- 1/2 teaspoon of aloe vera gel
- A clean mascara wand or cotton swab

Instructions:

1. In a small container, mix the castor oil and aloe vera gel until well combined.

2. Dip a clean mascara wand or cotton swab into the mixture.

3. Carefully apply to your eyelashes and eyebrows at night, being careful not to get any in your eyes.

4. Leave it on overnight and wash off with warm water in the morning.

5. Repeat nightly for best results.

These beginner-friendly DIY castor oil recipes are a great starting point for anyone looking to explore the benefits of this versatile oil. From promoting hair growth and skin health to aiding digestion and enhancing eyelash and eyebrow fullness, castor oil offers a wide range of natural remedies and beauty treatments that are easy to incorporate into your daily routine.

Simple Remedies for Skin and Hair

Harness the power of castor oil with these straightforward remedies designed to enhance the health and appearance of your skin and hair. Castor oil, rich in ricinoleic acid and omega-9 fatty acids, offers a natural solution for a variety of beauty concerns. These easy-to-follow recipes utilize castor oil's hydrating, anti-inflammatory, and antimicrobial properties to deliver noticeable results.

Hydrating Hair Mask for Dry and Brittle Hair

Materials:
- 3 tablespoons of castor oil
- 2 tablespoons of honey
- 1 egg (for extra protein)

Instructions:

1. Combine castor oil, honey, and the egg in a bowl. Mix thoroughly until you achieve a smooth consistency.

2. Apply the mixture to damp hair, focusing on the ends and working your way up to the scalp for an all-over treatment.

3. Cover your hair with a shower cap and let the mask sit for at least 30 minutes to allow the ingredients to penetrate deeply.

4. Rinse out the mask with lukewarm water and shampoo as usual. For best results, use this mask once a week to restore moisture and elasticity to your hair.

Soothing Skin Salve for Dry Patches and Eczema

Materials:
- 2 tablespoons of castor oil
- 2 tablespoons of coconut oil
- A few drops of lavender essential oil (for its calming and anti-inflammatory properties)

Instructions:

1. Gently melt the coconut oil in a double boiler or microwave, ensuring it's not too hot.

2. Stir in the castor oil and lavender essential oil until well combined.

3. Transfer the mixture to a clean jar and let it solidify. If in a hurry, you can place it in the refrigerator.

4. Apply a small amount of the salve to dry patches, eczema-prone areas, or anywhere your skin needs extra moisture. Use daily for best results.

Strengthening Scalp Treatment for Hair Growth

Materials:
- 4 tablespoons of castor oil
- 2 tablespoons of jojoba oil or olive oil (to thin out the castor oil and add additional nutrients)
- A few drops of peppermint essential oil (to stimulate the scalp)

Instructions:

1. In a small bowl, mix the castor oil with jojoba or olive oil. Add the peppermint essential oil and stir well.

2. Massage the oil blend into your scalp for several minutes, using circular motions to improve blood circulation.

3. Leave the treatment on for at least an hour or overnight for deep nourishment.

4. Wash your hair with a gentle shampoo and remove all the oil. Repeat once or twice a week to encourage hair growth and reduce hair fall.

Gentle Makeup Remover

Materials:
- 1 tablespoon of castor oil
- 2 tablespoons of almond oil or olive oil

Instructions:

1. Mix the castor oil with your choice of almond or olive oil in a small bottle. Shake well before each use.

2. Apply a small amount of the oil blend to a cotton pad or ball.

3. Gently wipe over your face to remove makeup. The oil mixture is especially effective at dissolving waterproof mascara and eyeliner.

4. Rinse your face with warm water and follow up with your regular cleanser.

These simple remedies leverage the natural benefits of castor oil to address common skin and hair issues. Incorporating castor oil into your beauty routine can lead to healthier, more vibrant skin and hair, showcasing the timeless beauty that comes from natural, nourishing ingredients.

Blending Castor Oil with Essential Oils

Combining castor oil with essential oils creates powerful synergies for skin, hair, and overall wellness. Castor oil's thick, nourishing properties make it an excellent carrier oil, enhancing the therapeutic benefits of essential oils. Here's how to blend castor oil with essential oils for specific health and beauty needs:

For Hair Growth and Scalp Health:

Materials:
- 2 tablespoons of castor oil
- 5 drops of rosemary essential oil
- 3 drops of peppermint essential oil

Instructions:

1. In a small bowl, mix the castor oil with rosemary and peppermint essential oils. Rosemary promotes hair growth and improves circulation, while peppermint stimulates the scalp, offering a refreshing sensation.

2. Massage the blend into your scalp for several minutes, focusing on areas of concern.

3. Leave the treatment on for at least 30 minutes or overnight for deep nourishment.

4. Wash your hair thoroughly with a gentle shampoo. Repeat 1-2 times a week.

For Soothing Dry, Irritated Skin:

Materials:
- 1 tablespoon of castor oil
- 4 drops of lavender essential oil
- 2 drops of chamomile essential oil

Instructions:

1. Combine castor oil with lavender and chamomile essential oils in a small container. Lavender offers calming properties, and chamomile soothes irritated skin.

2. Apply the mixture to dry, irritated areas, gently massaging until absorbed.

3. Use daily or as needed for relief and hydration.

For Acne-Prone Skin:

Materials:
- 1 tablespoon of castor oil
- 3 drops of tea tree essential oil
- 2 drops of lemon essential oil

Instructions:

1. Mix castor oil with tea tree and lemon essential oils. Tea tree is known for its antimicrobial and anti-inflammatory properties, making it ideal for acne-prone skin, while lemon helps to brighten and reduce scarring.

2. Apply a small amount of the blend to clean, affected areas using a cotton swab.

3. Use nightly, avoiding exposure to sunlight after application due to lemon oil's photosensitivity.

For Relaxation and Stress Relief:

Materials:
- 2 tablespoons of castor oil
- 5 drops of lavender essential oil
- 3 drops of frankincense essential oil

Instructions:

1. Blend castor oil with lavender and frankincense essential oils. Lavender aids in relaxation, and frankincense promotes a sense of peace and wellness.

2. Warm the oil mixture slightly for added comfort.

3. Massage into the shoulders, neck, and back or add to a warm bath for a soothing experience.

4. Use as needed to alleviate stress and unwind.

For Muscle and Joint Pain:

Materials:
- 2 tablespoons of castor oil
- 4 drops of eucalyptus essential oil
- 4 drops of ginger essential oil

Instructions:

1. Combine castor oil with eucalyptus and ginger essential oils. Eucalyptus provides cooling relief, while ginger warms and soothes sore muscles and joints.

2. Apply the oil blend to affected areas and massage gently.

3. Use after physical activity or whenever pain relief is needed.

When blending castor oil with essential oils, always perform a patch test to ensure no adverse reactions occur. Store any unused blends in a dark, glass bottle in a cool, dry place to maintain potency. By harnessing the combined power of castor oil and essential oils, you can create natural, effective remedies tailored to your specific health and beauty needs.

Infusing Castor Oil with Herbs for Added Benefits

Infusing castor oil with herbs amplifies its natural healing and beautifying properties, creating potent remedies for a variety of skin and hair concerns. This process involves steeping herbs in castor oil to extract their active compounds, resulting in an enriched oil that combines the benefits of both ingredients. Here's how to create your own herbal-infused castor oil at home.

Materials Needed:
- High-quality, cold-pressed castor oil
- Dried herbs of choice (e.g., rosemary for hair growth, lavender for relaxation, or chamomile for soothing

skin)
- Glass jar with a tight-fitting lid
- Cheesecloth or fine mesh strainer
- Dark glass bottle for storage

Step-by-Step Instructions:

1. Select Your Herbs: Choose one or more herbs based on the benefits you wish to achieve. For instance, rosemary can stimulate hair growth, lavender can reduce stress and improve skin health, and chamomile can soothe irritated skin.

2. Prepare the Jar: Fill a clean, dry glass jar about halfway with dried herbs. The herbs should be completely dry to prevent mold growth.

3. Add Castor Oil: Pour cold-pressed castor oil over the herbs, ensuring they are fully submerged. Fill the jar to within an inch of the top to allow for expansion.

4. Seal and Store: Tightly seal the jar and shake gently to mix the herbs and oil. Store the jar in a warm, sunny spot to facilitate infusion. A windowsill that receives plenty of sunlight is ideal.

5. Wait and Shake: Allow the mixture to infuse for 4-6 weeks, shaking the jar every few days to distribute the herbs and promote extraction.

6. Strain the Oil: After the infusion period, open the jar and strain the oil through cheesecloth or a fine mesh strainer into a clean bowl. Be sure to squeeze or press the herbs to extract as much oil as possible.

7. Transfer to Storage Bottle: Pour the strained oil into a dark glass bottle to protect it from light, which can degrade the oil's quality. Label the bottle with the contents and date of infusion.

8. Usage: Use your herbal-infused castor oil as a scalp treatment to promote hair growth, as a moisturizer for dry skin, or as a base for massage oils. The oil can be applied directly to the skin or hair, or added to homemade beauty products.

Safety Tips:
- Always perform a patch test before using the infused oil, especially if you've added new herbs you haven't used before.
- Ensure herbs are completely dry to avoid introducing moisture, which can lead to spoilage.
- Store the infused oil in a cool, dark place to preserve its potency.

Infusing castor oil with herbs not only boosts its inherent properties but also introduces the unique benefits of each herb, creating a versatile and powerful natural remedy. Whether you're aiming to enhance hair growth, soothe skin, or simply enjoy the aromatic benefits of herbs, herbal-infused castor oil is a valuable addition to your natural health and beauty toolkit.

Incorporating Castor Oil into Your Routine

Making castor oil a part of your daily or weekly routine can transform your approach to personal care, offering a natural, effective way to enhance your beauty and wellness practices. Here are practical ways to seamlessly integrate castor oil into your life, ensuring you reap its myriad benefits without disrupting your existing habits.

Morning Rituals:

Start your day with castor oil by adding it to your morning skincare routine. A few drops of castor oil can be mixed with your daily moisturizer to lock in hydration and protect your skin throughout the day. For hair care, consider massaging a small amount of castor oil into your scalp and hair ends while your hair is still damp from showering. This not only stimulates hair growth but also tames frizz and adds shine.

Evening Practices:

In the evening, castor oil can be your go-to for unwinding and treating your skin and hair to deep nourishment. Use it as a part of your double-cleansing process to remove makeup and impurities from the day. Follow up with a castor oil-enriched night cream to support skin repair and renewal as you sleep. For an intensive hair treatment, apply castor oil to your scalp and hair, wrap in a towel or shower cap, and leave it on overnight. This will provide ample time for the oil to penetrate deeply, promoting healthy hair growth and scalp health.

Weekly Indulgences:

Dedicate time each week for a castor oil pack, focusing on areas that need extra care, such as the abdomen for detoxification or sore joints and muscles for relief. This ritual not only supports physical wellness but also provides a moment of relaxation and self-care. Additionally, treat yourself to a weekly castor oil hair mask, blending it with ingredients like honey and egg for added conditioning, or simply use it on its own for its powerful effects.

On-the-Go Solutions:

For those with busy schedules, create a portable castor oil balm by mixing the oil with beeswax and storing it in a small jar. This balm can be used to hydrate lips, tame flyaway hairs, moisturize cuticles, or soothe dry skin patches throughout the day. Keep a small bottle of castor oil in your bag for quick touch-ups, ensuring you have a multipurpose beauty solution at your fingertips.

Integrating with Other Natural Remedies:

Enhance the efficacy of castor oil by combining it with other natural ingredients based on your specific needs. For instance, blend it with essential oils like lavender for relaxation or tea tree for its antimicrobial properties. You can also infuse castor oil with herbs like rosemary or chamomile to tailor it to your personal wellness goals.

By incorporating castor oil into your routine through these simple yet effective practices, you can harness its full potential to support your health, beauty, and well-being. Whether used alone or in combination with other natural ingredients, castor oil offers a versatile, powerful solution to many of today's wellness and beauty challenges.

Integrating Castor Oil into Your Morning and Evening Routines

Integrating Castor Oil into Your Morning and Evening Routines

Making castor oil a staple in both your morning and evening routines can significantly enhance your natural beauty regimen, providing nourishment and rejuvenation for your skin and hair. Here's how to seamlessly incorporate this versatile oil into your daily self-care practices.

Morning Routine:

- Hydrating Facial Moisturizer: Begin your day by mixing a few drops of castor oil with your regular facial moisturizer. This combination offers extra hydration, leaving your skin soft, supple, and ready to face the day. Apply it gently on your face and neck using upward strokes.

- Natural Eyelash Enhancer: Use a clean mascara brush to lightly apply castor oil to your eyelashes. This not only promotes growth but also adds a subtle gloss. Be careful to avoid direct contact with your eyes.

- Protective Hair Serum: Warm a small amount of castor oil between your palms and lightly run your hands through your hair, focusing on the ends. This acts as a protective barrier against environmental damage and helps control frizz throughout the day.

Evening Routine:

- Deep Cleansing Oil: Castor oil's thick consistency makes it an excellent choice for an oil cleansing method in the evening. Massage a generous amount onto your dry face to dissolve makeup, dirt, and impurities from the day. Wipe away with a warm, damp cloth for a deep clean that leaves your skin balanced and nourished.

- Overnight Hair Treatment: For an intensive hair conditioning treatment, massage a mixture of castor oil and a lighter carrier oil, like almond or jojoba, into your scalp and hair before bed. Wrap your hair in a towel or a shower cap. This treatment promotes hair growth, moisturizes the scalp, and repairs split ends. Wash your hair in the morning with a gentle shampoo.

- Cuticle and Nail Care: Rub a small amount of castor oil into your cuticles and nails each night. Its rich nutrients strengthen nails and moisturize cuticles, promoting healthy nail growth and preventing brittleness.

Weekly Additions:

- Scalp Detox Mask: Once a week, treat your scalp to a detoxifying mask by mixing castor oil with bentonite clay and apple cider vinegar. Apply the mixture to your scalp for 15-20 minutes before rinsing. This mask helps to remove buildup, soothe the scalp, and promote healthy hair growth.

- Soothing Bath Additive: Add a few tablespoons of castor oil to your bath water once a week for a luxurious, skin-softening soak. The oil's fatty acids soothe dry skin, while its warmth and natural fragrance offer a relaxing experience.

Incorporating castor oil into your morning and evening routines is a simple yet effective way to leverage its myriad benefits for your skin and hair. With consistent use, you'll notice improvements in hydration, growth, and overall health, making castor oil a valuable addition to your natural beauty arsenal.

Quick Castor Oil Hacks for Busy Schedules

For those juggling a packed schedule, finding time for elaborate beauty and wellness routines can be a challenge. However, incorporating castor oil into your daily life doesn't have to be time-consuming. Here are some quick and effective castor oil hacks that can easily fit into even the busiest schedules, ensuring you don't miss out on the benefits of this versatile oil.

- Morning Eyelash and Eyebrow Boost: Dip a clean mascara wand or a cotton swab in castor oil and swiftly apply to your eyelashes and eyebrows while waiting for your morning coffee to brew. This not only promotes growth but also keeps them well-groomed throughout the day.

- Castor Oil Face Wipes: Pre-soak a few cotton pads in a mixture of castor oil and your favorite skin-friendly oil, such as almond or jojoba oil. Store them in a sealed container. In the morning or night, grab a pad for a quick facial cleanse or makeup remover that moisturizes and cleanses simultaneously.

- Quick Cuticle Care: Keep a small bottle of castor oil at your desk or in your purse. During a brief moment of downtime, massage a drop into your cuticles to keep them hydrated and prevent hangnails.

- Overnight Hair Treatment Shortcut: If you don't have time for a lengthy hair mask session, simply apply castor oil to the ends of your hair before bed. Tie your hair up and cover your pillow with an old towel to protect your linens. This minimal effort treatment does wonders for split ends and overall hair texture with zero daytime commitment.

- On-the-Go Scalp Treatment: For a quick scalp boost, mix castor oil with a few drops of peppermint oil in a roller bottle. During the day, roll directly onto your scalp along the hairline or any area needing attention. The peppermint oil provides a refreshing sensation, while the castor oil works to moisturize and promote hair health.

- Speedy Detox Bath: Add 1-2 tablespoons of castor oil to your bathwater along with Epsom salts and a few drops of lavender oil for a detoxifying and relaxing soak. This quick addition takes no extra time but enhances your bath's health benefits.

- Instant Lip Balm: For chapped lips, apply a tiny dab of castor oil directly to your lips. Its thick consistency provides long-lasting hydration, perfect for dry, busy days when you can't constantly reapply lip balm.

- Castor Oil Hand Treatment: Before driving, massage a few drops of castor oil into your hands, especially if you have a long commute. The warmth of the car helps the oil absorb, and you'll arrive with soft, moisturized hands without taking any additional time out of your day.

These hacks demonstrate that even the busiest individuals can incorporate the nourishing benefits of castor oil into their daily routines. By choosing multitasking methods and quick applications, you can enjoy the myriad advantages of castor oil without compromising your schedule.

Travel-Friendly Castor Oil Solutions

For the modern, health-conscious woman on the go, maintaining a natural beauty and wellness routine while traveling can be a challenge. Castor oil, with its versatile applications for skin, hair, and overall health, is a must-have item in your travel kit. Here are practical, travel-friendly castor oil solutions that are easy to pack, comply with travel regulations, and ensure you can continue your natural health regimen no matter where you are.

- Mini Castor Oil Bottles: Transfer castor oil into small, leak-proof bottles that comply with airline regulations for liquids. This ensures you can carry castor oil in your carry-on luggage without any hassle. A 100ml (3.4 oz) bottle is typically within the limit and perfect for short trips.

- Pre-Made Castor Oil Packs: Prepare a few castor oil packs in advance by soaking pieces of cloth in castor oil, then sealing them in zip-lock bags. This way, you can easily use them for detoxification or pain relief without having to carry the entire bottle. Simply warm them up with a hotel room hairdryer or in a warm bath before use.

- Castor Oil Capsules: For internal health benefits, such as digestive support, consider packing castor oil capsules. They are convenient, mess-free, and easy to dose, making them ideal for travelers looking to maintain or address specific health concerns while away from home.

- DIY Castor Oil Wipes: Create your own castor oil wipes by soaking cotton pads in castor oil and storing them in a sealed bag. These wipes can be a lifesaver for removing makeup, hydrating dry skin, or quick hair touch-ups, offering a compact and convenient solution.

- Solid Castor Oil Balm: Combine castor oil with beeswax and coconut oil to create a solid balm that's travel-friendly and won't spill in your bag. This balm can be used to moisturize lips, skin, and cuticles, tame eyebrows, and even as a hair end protector against split ends.

- Travel-Sized Hair and Scalp Treatment Kit: Mix castor oil with your favorite essential oils and store in a small dropper bottle for an easy-to-apply hair and scalp treatment. This kit can fit in any bag, ensuring you can keep your hair routine consistent, promoting growth and shine even while traveling.

- Castor Oil Eye Serum Roller: For a refreshing under-eye treatment that combats puffiness and dark circles, fill a small roller bottle with castor oil. Its compact size makes it perfect for refreshing your eyes during long flights or after a day of sightseeing.

By incorporating these travel-friendly castor oil solutions into your packing list, you can ensure that your commitment to natural health and beauty doesn't take a vacation when you do. These simple, effective strategies allow you to enjoy the benefits of castor oil wherever your travels may take you, keeping your skin glowing, your hair lustrous, and your body healthy without compromising on convenience or luggage space.

Book 3: Castor Oil for Radiant Skin

Achieving Clear and Glowing Skin

Castor oil, a natural humectant, draws moisture from the air into the skin, making it an excellent choice for maintaining hydrated and glowing skin. Its unique composition, rich in ricinoleic acid, offers anti-inflammatory benefits, reducing redness and blemishes. For those seeking a radiant complexion, incorporating castor oil into your skincare routine can yield significant results. Here's how:

Castor Oil Cleansing Method for Acne-Prone Skin

Materials:
- 1 tablespoon of castor oil
- 2 tablespoons of jojoba oil

Instructions:

1. Mix castor oil with jojoba oil in a clean container. The jojoba oil dilutes the castor oil, making it easier to spread and ensuring it doesn't clog pores.

2. Gently massage the oil mixture onto your dry face for a couple of minutes. This process helps to lift and dissolve impurities, makeup, and excess oil from the pores.

3. Soak a clean washcloth in hot water, wring out the excess, and place it over your face. The steam will help open the pores, allowing the oils to penetrate deeply.

4. Once the washcloth cools, use it to gently wipe away the oil. Rinse the cloth and repeat if necessary.

5. Finish by rinsing your face with cool water to close the pores. Pat dry with a clean towel.

Anti-Aging Face Serum: Wrinkles and Fine Lines

Materials:
- 2 tablespoons of castor oil
- 2 tablespoons of sweet almond oil
- 5 drops of vitamin E oil
- 5 drops of lavender essential oil

Instructions:

1. Combine all ingredients in a dark glass dropper bottle and shake well to blend.

2. Each night, after cleansing, apply 2-3 drops of the serum to your face and neck, focusing on areas with fine lines and wrinkles.

3. Gently massage in upward motions until fully absorbed. The serum works overnight to promote cell regeneration and improve skin elasticity.

Castor Oil Masks for an Instant Glow

Materials:
- 1 tablespoon of castor oil
- 1 tablespoon of honey
- 1 egg white

Instructions:

1. In a small bowl, whisk together castor oil, honey, and egg white until you achieve a smooth consistency.

2. Apply the mask evenly over your clean face, avoiding the eye area.

3. Leave the mask on for 15-20 minutes, allowing the ingredients to nourish and revitalize the skin.

4. Rinse off with warm water, followed by a splash of cold water to tighten the pores. Pat dry and follow up with your regular moisturizer.

Treating Specific Skin Issues with Castor Oil

Castor oil's healing properties extend beyond basic skincare, offering solutions for specific skin issues such as eczema, psoriasis, and dry skin. Its ability to penetrate deeply into the skin makes it an effective treatment for these conditions.

Eczema, Psoriasis, and Dry Skin Solutions

For eczema and psoriasis, the anti-inflammatory and moisturizing properties of castor oil can alleviate discomfort and reduce flakiness. Apply a small amount of castor oil directly to affected areas before bed, covering with a soft cloth or bandage to protect your linens. For dry skin, mix castor oil with coconut oil for an extra hydrating lotion, applying it to your body while still slightly damp from a shower to lock in moisture.

Scar and Stretch Mark Reduction

The fatty acids in castor oil promote the growth of healthy skin tissue, making it beneficial for reducing the appearance of scars and stretch marks. Regularly massage a mixture of castor oil and rosehip oil onto scars or stretch marks to gradually fade their appearance and improve skin texture.

Healing Sunburns and Skin Discoloration

Castor oil can soothe sunburned skin, reducing inflammation and peeling. Apply a thin layer of castor oil to the affected area, allowing its healing properties to restore damaged skin. For skin discoloration, consistent application of castor oil can help even out skin tone over time, thanks to its ability to penetrate deeply and encourage the regeneration of skin cells.

Castor Oil for Lips, Nails, and More

Nourishing Lip Balms and Treatment

For chapped lips, a simple balm made from castor oil and beeswax can provide lasting hydration and protection. Melt equal parts of castor oil and beeswax together, pour into small containers, and let cool. Apply to your lips as needed for a smooth, soft finish.

Strengthening Nails and Cuticles

Mix castor oil with a few drops of lemon essential oil and apply to your nails and cuticles nightly. This treatment strengthens nails, prevents fungal infections, and keeps cuticles soft and manageable.

Castor Oil for Smoother, Hydrated Hands

Create a hand treatment by mixing castor oil with shea butter and aloe vera gel. Apply this mixture to your hands at night, wearing cotton gloves to enhance absorption. Wake up to softer, more hydrated skin, ready to tackle the day.

By integrating castor oil into your skincare routine, you can address a wide range of skin concerns, from daily care to specific treatments. Its natural, healing properties make castor oil a versatile and effective choice for achieving and maintaining radiant skin.

Achieving Clear and Glowing Skin

Castor oil, renowned for its hydrating and anti-inflammatory properties, is a secret weapon for those aiming to achieve clear and glowing skin. Its high content of ricinoleic acid not only combats acne-causing bacteria but also soothes irritated skin, making it a versatile solution for a variety of skin concerns. Here's how to harness the power of castor oil for radiant skin:

Deep Cleansing with Castor Oil

Castor oil's thick consistency allows it to deeply penetrate pores, pulling out impurities and excess oil that can lead to breakouts. To use castor oil as a deep cleanser:

1. Mix equal parts of castor oil with a carrier oil like jojoba or sweet almond oil to create a blend that is easier to spread on your skin.

2. Gently massage the oil blend onto your dry face for a few minutes, focusing on areas prone to blackheads and acne.

3. Soak a clean washcloth in hot water, wring out the excess, and place it over your face. The steam will help open your pores, allowing the castor oil to work more effectively.

4. Once the washcloth cools, use it to gently wipe away the oil. Repeat if necessary, then splash your face with cold water to close the pores.

Moisturizing for Soft, Supple Skin

Despite its ability to cleanse deeply, castor oil is also an excellent moisturizer. Its humectant properties help lock moisture into the skin:

1. After cleansing, while your skin is still damp, take a few drops of castor oil on your fingertips.

2. Warm the oil by rubbing your fingers together, then gently press it onto your face, focusing on dry areas or fine lines.

3. Allow the oil to absorb fully before applying makeup or sunscreen.

Treating Acne and Blemishes

The antibacterial properties of castor oil make it effective in treating acne and reducing blemishes:

1. Cleanse your face thoroughly using the deep cleansing method mentioned above.

2. Dab a small amount of castor oil directly onto blemishes using a clean finger or cotton swab.

3. Leave it on overnight, and rinse off in the morning with warm water.

4. For best results, incorporate this into your nightly skincare routine.

Soothing Inflammation and Reducing Scars

Castor oil can also help reduce inflammation and the appearance of scars:

1. Mix castor oil with a healing oil like rosehip seed oil, known for its scar-reducing properties.

2. Apply the mixture to areas of concern, gently massaging in circular motions to promote blood flow and healing.

3. Use consistently every night for noticeable improvement in skin texture and scar appearance.

Brightening the Under-Eye Area

To address dark circles and under-eye puffiness:

1. Before bed, apply a small amount of castor oil to your under-eye area with your ring finger, tapping gently to encourage absorption.

2. Be careful not to apply too close to the eyes to avoid irritation.

3. In the morning, rinse your face with cool water to reduce puffiness and reveal a brighter, more refreshed eye area.

By incorporating castor oil into your skincare regimen, you can achieve clear, glowing skin that radiates health and vitality. Its natural, healing properties work to cleanse, moisturize, and repair the skin, making castor oil a must-have in your beauty arsenal.

Castor Oil Cleansing Method for Acne-Prone Skin

Acne-prone skin requires a gentle yet effective cleansing routine to remove impurities without stripping the skin of its natural oils. The castor oil cleansing method leverages the potent anti-inflammatory and antibacterial properties of castor oil to cleanse, soothe, and heal acne-prone skin. Here's a step-by-step guide to incorporating this method into your skincare routine:

Materials Needed:
- Castor oil
- Carrier oil (such as jojoba oil, grapeseed oil, or sweet almond oil)
- Soft washcloth
- Hot water

Instructions:

1. Prepare Your Oil Blend: The key to the castor oil cleansing method is to find the right balance be-

tween castor oil and a carrier oil. For acne-prone skin, a recommended starting ratio is one part castor oil to three parts carrier oil. Adjust the ratio based on your skin's response; more castor oil for oilier skin and less for dry skin.

2. Apply the Oil: Pour a generous amount of the oil blend into the palm of your hand. Rub your hands together to warm the oil and then gently massage it into your face. Spend a couple of minutes massaging the oil in circular motions, focusing on areas with congestion or breakouts. This massage helps the oil penetrate the pores and dissolve impurities, makeup, and excess sebum.

3. Steam Your Face: Soak the washcloth in hot water, wring out the excess water, and then drape it over your face. The steam will help open the pores, allowing the castor oil to draw out impurities. Leave the washcloth on until it cools to room temperature.

4. Wipe Away the Oil: Use the same washcloth to gently wipe away the oil from your face. You may need to rinse the washcloth and repeat this step to ensure all oil is removed. Be gentle to avoid irritating the skin.

5. Rinse and Dry: Splash your face with cool water to rinse away any remaining oil and help close the pores. Pat your face dry with a clean towel.

6. Moisturize If Needed: Depending on your skin type, you may or may not need to apply a moisturizer after cleansing. If your skin feels tight or dry, apply a small amount of your preferred moisturizer or a few drops of your carrier oil.

Benefits and Tips:
- Deep Cleansing: This method deeply cleanses the pores without stripping the skin's natural barrier, reducing the occurrence of acne breakouts.
- Balancing Oil Production: Castor oil helps regulate sebum production, which can prevent future breakouts.
- Healing Properties: The anti-inflammatory properties of castor oil can reduce redness and swelling associated with acne.

For best results, use the castor oil cleansing method in the evening to remove the day's buildup of impurities. Start with 2-3 times a week and adjust based on how your skin responds. This method can be a game-changer for acne-prone skin, offering a natural and effective way to achieve clearer, healthier-looking skin.

Anti-Aging Face Serum: Wrinkles and Fine Lines

Creating an anti-aging face serum using castor oil is a natural and effective way to combat wrinkles and fine lines. This serum leverages the hydrating and healing properties of castor oil, combined with other natural oils known for their anti-aging benefits. Here's how to make your own:

Materials Needed:
- 2 tablespoons of castor oil
- 2 tablespoons of sweet almond oil
- 5 drops of vitamin E oil
- 5 drops of lavender essential oil
- Dark glass dropper bottle

Instructions:

1. Combine Oils: In a clean bowl, mix the castor oil and sweet almond oil. These oils serve as the base of your serum, providing deep moisturization and smoothing the skin's texture.

2. Add Vitamin E and Lavender Oil: Add the vitamin E oil to the mixture. Vitamin E is a powerful antioxidant that can help protect the skin from damage caused by free radicals and UV exposure. Then, add the lavender essential oil, which not only adds a calming scent but also offers additional skin-soothing and regenerative properties.

3. Transfer to Dropper Bottle: Carefully pour your serum mixture into a dark glass dropper bottle. The dark glass helps protect the oils from light, preserving their potency.

4. Application: To use, cleanse your face thoroughly and pat dry. Apply 2-3 drops of the serum to your fingertips and gently massage into your face and neck, focusing on areas with visible wrinkles and fine lines. The serum can be used nightly as part of your skincare routine.

5. Storage: Store your anti-aging serum in a cool, dark place to maintain its efficacy. The shelf life of your homemade serum is approximately 6 months.

Benefits:
- Moisturizing: Castor oil deeply hydrates the skin, reducing the appearance of wrinkles and preventing the formation of new fine lines.
- Healing: The ricinoleic acid in castor oil promotes the growth of healthy skin tissue, aiding in the repair of damaged skin.
- Antioxidant Protection: Vitamin E provides antioxidant protection, helping to ward off skin damage from environmental stressors.
- Soothing: Lavender essential oil calms the skin, reducing redness and inflammation.

By incorporating this DIY anti-aging face serum into your nightly skincare routine, you can enjoy the benefits of castor oil along with the synergistic effects of sweet almond oil, vitamin E, and lavender essential oil. Together, these ingredients work to nourish, protect, and rejuvenate your skin, helping to maintain a youthful and radiant complexion.

Castor Oil Masks for an Instant Glow

For an instant glow that leaves your skin feeling rejuvenated and looking radiant, a castor oil mask is your go-to solution. This mask combines the hydrating and anti-inflammatory benefits of castor oil with other natural ingredients to create a powerful, glow-inducing treatment. Here's how to whip up this simple yet effective mask:

Materials:
- 1 tablespoon of castor oil
- 1 tablespoon of raw honey- 1 ripe banana

Instructions:

1. Mash the Banana: Start by mashing the ripe banana in a small bowl until you achieve a smooth consistency. Bananas are rich in vitamins and antioxidants, which help to moisturize the skin and reduce the appearance of fine lines and wrinkles.

2. Mix in Honey and Castor Oil: Add the tablespoon of raw honey and the tablespoon of castor oil to the mashed banana. Honey is a natural humectant that draws moisture into the skin, while castor oil works to reduce inflammation and promote healthy skin regeneration.

3. Apply the Mask: Once all the ingredients are thoroughly mixed, apply the mask evenly over your clean face. Be sure to avoid the eye area to prevent irritation.

4. Relax and Wait: Leave the mask on for about 15 to 20 minutes. This is the perfect time to relax and let the mask do its work. The natural ingredients will penetrate deep into your skin, providing hydration, reducing inflammation, and leaving you with a natural glow.

5. Rinse Off: After the time is up, rinse the mask off with lukewarm water. Gently pat your face dry with a soft towel.

6. Moisturize: Follow up with your favorite moisturizer to lock in the hydration and benefits of the mask.

Benefits:
- Instant Hydration: This mask delivers an intense hydration boost to your skin, thanks to the moisturizing properties of both castor oil and honey.
- Glowing Complexion: The combination of ingredients works to brighten the complexion, leaving your skin with a natural, healthy glow.
- Soothes Inflammation: Castor oil's anti-inflammatory properties help to calm irritated skin, making this

mask ideal for those with sensitive or acne-prone skin types.
- Anti-Aging Effects: Regular use of this mask can help to reduce the signs of aging, thanks to the antioxidants found in bananas and honey, which fight free radical damage.

For best results, incorporate this castor oil mask into your skincare routine once or twice a week. Over time, you'll notice a significant improvement in your skin's texture, hydration, and overall radiance. This simple, natural remedy is a powerful addition to your beauty arsenal, harnessing the ancient secrets of castor oil to help you achieve timeless beauty.

Treating Specific Skin Issues with Castor Oil

Castor oil, with its rich content of ricinoleic acid, offers a natural remedy for a variety of specific skin issues, including eczema, psoriasis, and acne. Its anti-inflammatory, antimicrobial, and moisturizing properties make it an excellent choice for those seeking to soothe irritated skin, reduce redness, and promote healing. Here, we explore how to use castor oil effectively for these conditions, providing relief and improving skin health.

Eczema Relief with Castor Oil

Eczema, characterized by itchy, inflamed, and dry skin, can be significantly soothed with regular applications of castor oil. Its hydrating properties help to lock in moisture, reducing dryness and flakiness.
- Application: Gently apply a thin layer of pure, cold-pressed castor oil to the affected areas. For enhanced absorption, do this after a warm bath or shower when the skin is still moist. Cover the area with a soft cloth or bandage overnight to allow the oil to deeply penetrate the skin. Repeat nightly until symptoms improve.

Psoriasis Treatment

Psoriasis sufferers can benefit from castor oil's ability to soften scales, ease itching, and reduce inflammation.
- Method: Mix equal parts of castor oil with a carrier oil, such as coconut oil, to create a soothing blend. Apply this mixture to the scaly patches before bedtime. Wrap the area with plastic wrap and cover it with a warm cloth to enhance penetration. In the morning, gently cleanse the area. Use daily for best results.

Acne and Blemish Control

The antimicrobial properties of castor oil make it effective in combating acne-causing bacteria, while its anti-inflammatory benefits help to reduce the size and redness of pimples.
- Spot Treatment: After cleansing your face, apply a small amount of castor oil directly onto blemishes with a clean cotton swab. Leave it on overnight and rinse off in the morning. For a more intensive treat-

ment, create a mask by mixing castor oil with turmeric powder to form a paste, apply to the entire face or affected areas, leave for 15-20 minutes, then rinse off. Use 2-3 times a week.

Scar Reduction

Regular use of castor oil can improve the appearance of scars by promoting the growth of healthier skin tissue and keeping the area moisturized.
- Routine: Mix castor oil with a few drops of lavender essential oil, known for its skin-healing properties. Massage this blend into the scarred area for several minutes each night, using circular motions to encourage blood flow. Consistency is key for visible results.

Soothing Sunburn

Castor oil can also provide relief for sunburned skin, thanks to its anti-inflammatory properties and ability to restore moisture.
- After-Sun Care: Combine castor oil with aloe vera gel, an excellent natural remedy for sunburn, in equal parts. Apply generously to the sunburned area. The mixture will soothe the burn, reduce inflammation, and prevent peeling.

By incorporating castor oil into your skincare regimen, you can naturally address and manage these common skin issues. Its versatility and safety profile make it a valuable addition to any natural beauty and wellness toolkit. Remember, while castor oil is generally safe for topical use, it's always recommended to perform a patch test before applying it to larger areas of the skin, especially for those with sensitive skin or allergies.

Eczema, Psoriasis, and Dry Skin Solutions

Eczema, psoriasis, and chronic dry skin conditions can be both uncomfortable and challenging to manage. The anti-inflammatory and deeply moisturizing properties of castor oil make it an excellent natural remedy for soothing these skin issues. Here's how to use castor oil to alleviate symptoms and promote healthier skin.

For Eczema:

Eczema sufferers often struggle with dry, itchy, and inflamed skin. Castor oil's hydration capabilities can provide much-needed relief.
- Application: Gently warm a small amount of pure, cold-pressed castor oil by rubbing it between your hands. Apply a thin layer to the affected areas. For best results, do this at night, allowing the oil to work while you sleep. Cover the area with a soft, breathable fabric to protect your bedding.

For Psoriasis:

The buildup of skin cells associated with psoriasis can lead to scaling, itching, and thick patches of skin. Castor oil can help soften these areas and reduce inflammation.
- Treatment: Mix castor oil with a carrier oil like coconut oil to thin its consistency. Apply this blend to the patches of psoriasis before bed. Wrap the area lightly with plastic wrap to keep the oil in place and maximize absorption. Wash off in the morning with a gentle cleanser.

For Dry Skin:

Dry skin lacks moisture and can feel tight and uncomfortable. Castor oil acts as a natural humectant, pulling moisture into the skin and locking it in.
- Moisturizer: After showering, while your skin is still damp, apply a mixture of castor oil and your favorite moisturizer. Focus on particularly dry areas such as elbows, knees, and heels. The oil will seal in the moisture from your shower, leaving your skin soft and supple.

Additional Tips:
- Frequency: Start with applying castor oil to your skin 2-3 times a week. Depending on your skin's tolerance and the severity of your condition, you may adjust the frequency.
- Patch Test: Always perform a patch test on a small area of your skin before applying castor oil widely, especially if you have sensitive skin.
- Quality Matters: Use only high-quality, cold-pressed, organic castor oil to ensure you're applying the purest form to your delicate skin.
- Hydration: Drink plenty of water throughout the day to help your skin stay hydrated from the inside out. This is especially important when treating dry skin conditions.

By incorporating castor oil into your skincare routine, you can naturally soothe and manage the symptoms of eczema, psoriasis, and dry skin. Its healing properties not only address the discomfort associated with these conditions but also promote the regeneration of healthy skin cells, offering a gentle and effective solution for those seeking relief from chronic skin issues.

Scar and Stretch Mark Reduction

The natural healing properties of castor oil make it an effective remedy for reducing the appearance of scars and stretch marks. Its rich content of ricinoleic acid, an unsaturated omega-9 fatty acid, promotes the growth of healthy skin tissue and improves skin elasticity, which can minimize the look of both new and old scars and stretch marks. Here's a step-by-step guide to using castor oil for scar and stretch mark reduction:

Materials Needed:
- Pure, cold-pressed castor oil
- Clean, soft cloth or cotton ball

- Plastic wrap (optional for scars)
- Warm compress or heating pad (optional)

Instructions:

1. Clean the Area: Start with clean skin. Gently wash the area with mild soap and water, then pat dry with a soft towel.

2. Apply Castor Oil: Take a small amount of castor oil on your fingertips or a cotton ball. Apply a thin layer of oil over the scar or stretch marks. For scars, you can use a bit more oil to thoroughly cover the area.

3. Massage: Gently massage the oil into the skin using circular motions. This helps to increase blood flow to the area, which can aid in healing. Spend a few minutes massaging the oil to ensure it's well absorbed.

4. For Scars - Apply Warm Compress: (Optional) After massaging the oil into a scar, cover the area with a clean cloth and apply a warm compress or heating pad for 20-30 minutes. The warmth helps to further penetrate the skin. For stretch marks, this step can be skipped.

5. Cover: (Optional for overnight treatment) If you're treating scars, you can cover the area with plastic wrap after applying the oil to keep the oil in contact with the skin for an extended period. For stretch marks, wear comfortable, breathable clothing that won't absorb the oil.

6. Leave On: For best results, leave the castor oil on the skin for several hours or overnight. This allows the oil ample time to penetrate and promote healing.

7. Rinse Off: Wash the area with warm water and mild soap. Pat dry gently.

8. Repeat: For effective results, repeat this process daily. Consistency is key when it comes to reducing the appearance of scars and stretch marks.

Tips for Success:
- Patience is Essential: Improvement takes time. Regular use over several weeks to months is necessary to see significant changes.
- Stay Hydrated: Drinking plenty of water helps to keep your skin hydrated and enhances the oil's effectiveness.
- Healthy Diet: A diet rich in vitamins and minerals supports skin health and can aid the healing process.
- Sun Protection: Protecting your skin from the sun is crucial, as UV exposure can darken scars and stretch marks, making them more noticeable.

By following these steps, you can harness the power of castor oil to improve the appearance of scars and stretch marks, promoting smoother, more supple skin. Remember, while castor oil is a natural and effective remedy, results vary from person to person, and patience and consistency are key to achieving the best outcomes.

Healing Sunburns and Skin Discoloration

Sunburns and skin discoloration can be both uncomfortable and aesthetically displeasing, presenting a challenge for those seeking to maintain an even and healthy skin tone. Castor oil, with its anti-inflammatory and healing properties, offers a natural remedy to soothe sunburned skin and address areas of discoloration. Here's how to use castor oil effectively for these specific skin concerns.

Soothing Sunburns with Castor Oil:

1. Cool the Skin: Before applying castor oil, it's important to cool the sunburned area with a damp cloth or take a cool bath to reduce heat and inflammation.
2. Apply Castor Oil Gently: Once the skin is cooled, lightly apply a thin layer of cold-pressed castor oil to the sunburned area. Its anti-inflammatory properties help soothe the skin and reduce redness.

3. Cover with a Soft Cloth: If possible, cover the treated area with a soft, lightweight cloth to protect the skin and help the oil absorb more effectively.

4. Reapply as Needed: For severe sunburns, reapply castor oil 2-3 times a day until symptoms improve. Its hydrating properties will prevent peeling and aid in the skin's healing process.

Addressing Skin Discoloration:

Skin discoloration, including dark spots and uneven skin tones, can be gradually lightened with regular application of castor oil.

1. Cleanse the Skin: Start with a clean face or area of skin where discoloration is present. Gently pat dry after washing.

2. Apply Castor Oil to Discolored Areas: Using a cotton swab or your fingertips, apply castor oil directly to dark spots or uneven skin tones each night. The fatty acids in castor oil can help to fade discoloration over time by promoting the growth of healthy skin cells.

3. Massage Gently: For better absorption, softly massage the area for a few minutes. This also increases blood circulation, which aids in the healing process.

4. Leave Overnight: Allow the castor oil to work its magic overnight. In the morning, rinse your face with lukewarm water and follow up with your regular skincare routine.

5. Protect from the Sun: To prevent further discoloration, apply sunscreen daily. UV exposure can worsen skin discoloration and counteract the benefits of castor oil.

Consistency is Key:

For both sunburn treatment and correcting skin discoloration, consistency in application is crucial. While castor oil is gentle and effective, results will vary based on the severity of the condition and individual skin types. Continued use over several weeks to months is often necessary to see significant improvements.

Patch Test:

Always perform a patch test before using castor oil extensively, especially on sensitive or damaged skin, to ensure there is no adverse reaction.

By incorporating castor oil into your skincare regimen for sunburn relief and to address skin discoloration, you can harness its natural, healing properties to maintain a healthy, even complexion.

Castor Oil for Lips, Nails, and More

Castor oil, a versatile and deeply nourishing natural oil, is not just for skin and hair—it's also a miracle worker for lips, nails, and more. Its rich composition, primarily of ricinoleic acid, makes it an excellent choice for providing moisture, promoting growth, and enhancing the overall health of these often-neglected areas. Here's how to incorporate castor oil into your care routine for lips, nails, and beyond.

Nourishing Lip Balms and Treatment

Chapped lips can benefit greatly from the hydrating properties of castor oil. To create a simple yet effective lip balm:
- Mix 1 tablespoon of castor oil with 1 tablespoon of beeswax and ½ tablespoon of honey.
- Melt the mixture in a double boiler, stirring until well combined.
- Pour into small lip balm containers and allow to cool and solidify.
- Apply to your lips as needed for instant hydration and protection against the elements.

This balm can also be used as an overnight lip treatment. Simply apply a thicker layer before bed, and wake up to soft, supple lips.

Strengthening Nails and Cuticles

For stronger nails and softer cuticles, castor oil is a go-to solution:

- Before bed, apply a small amount of castor oil directly to each nail and cuticle.
- Massage gently for a few minutes to increase absorption and stimulate blood flow to the area.
- Wear cotton gloves overnight to lock in moisture and protect your linens.
- Repeat nightly for best results, and watch as your nails become stronger and your cuticles more supple.

Castor Oil for Smoother, Hydrated Hands

Dry hands can also reap the benefits of castor oil's moisturizing properties:
- Combine equal parts of castor oil and your favorite hand cream for an intensive moisture treatment.
- Apply generously to your hands, paying special attention to dry areas and knuckles.
- For an added boost, wear cotton gloves for an hour or overnight, allowing the mixture to deeply penetrate and hydrate the skin.

Eyebrow and Eyelash Growth

Thin eyebrows and eyelashes can be thickened with regular application of castor oil:
- Using a clean mascara wand or cotton swab, apply castor oil to your eyebrows and lashes at night.
- Be careful to avoid getting oil into your eyes.
- Consistent use can lead to thicker, fuller brows and lashes over time.

Soothing Dry Elbows and Heels

Rough, dry patches on elbows and heels can be softened with castor oil:
- Apply castor oil directly to these areas after showering, when the skin is still damp.
- Massage in thoroughly until the oil is absorbed.
- For deep treatment, cover the area with a warm cloth for 20-30 minutes or wear socks overnight if treating heels.

Enhancing Homemade Beauty Products

Castor oil can also be a valuable addition to DIY beauty products, such as:
- Adding a few drops to homemade face masks for extra hydration.
- Incorporating it into homemade hair masks for added strength and shine.
- Using it as a base for homemade soaps for its moisturizing properties.

Incorporating castor oil into your routine for lips, nails, and more not only enhances the beauty and health of these areas but also leverages the oil's natural, healing properties for overall wellness. Its versatility and efficacy make castor oil a staple in any natural beauty and health regimen.

Nourishing Lip Balms and Treatment

Creating your own nourishing lip balm with castor oil is a simple and effective way to combat dry, chapped lips. Castor oil, known for its deep moisturizing properties, can provide a protective barrier that seals in moisture and promotes healing. This DIY lip balm recipe combines castor oil with other natural ingredients to create a soothing and hydrating treatment for your lips.

Materials Needed:
- 2 tablespoons of castor oil
- 1 tablespoon of beeswax pellets
- 1 tablespoon of coconut oil
- 5 drops of vitamin E oil (optional for added nourishment)
- 5 drops of your choice of essential oil (peppermint or lavender work well for a soothing effect)
- Small lip balm tubes or tins for storage

Instructions:

1. Melt the Beeswax and Coconut Oil: In a double boiler or a glass bowl over simmering water, melt the beeswax and coconut oil together. Stir continuously until completely melted and combined.

2. Add Castor Oil: Once the beeswax and coconut oil are melted, remove from heat and stir in the castor oil. Mix thoroughly to ensure all ingredients are well combined.

3. Incorporate Vitamin E and Essential Oils: Add the vitamin E oil and your chosen essential oil to the mixture. Vitamin E acts as an antioxidant that can help extend the shelf life of your lip balm, while essential oils provide a pleasant scent and additional therapeutic benefits.

4. Pour into Containers: Carefully pour the liquid mixture into your lip balm tubes or tins. Fill each container to just below the top to prevent spilling as the mixture solidifies.

5. Let Cool: Allow the lip balm to cool and solidify completely. This may take a few hours at room temperature. You can also place them in the refrigerator to speed up the process.

6. Cap and Label: Once solid, you can cap the containers and label them. Your homemade lip balm is now ready to use or give as a thoughtful, natural gift.

Usage Tips:
- Apply to your lips as often as needed, especially before exposure to harsh weather conditions to prevent drying and cracking.
- For an extra glossy finish, apply a small amount of pure castor oil over the lip balm.
- If your lips are severely chapped, gently exfoliate with a soft toothbrush or sugar scrub before applying the lip balm for better absorption.

This DIY nourishing lip balm harnesses the hydrating power of castor oil, combined with the protective qualities of beeswax and the moisturizing benefits of coconut oil, to provide a natural remedy for dry, chapped lips. With regular use, your lips will feel softer, smoother, and more resilient against the elements.

Strengthening Nails and Cuticles

Strengthening Nails and Cuticles

For healthier, stronger nails and softer, more resilient cuticles, incorporating castor oil into your nail care routine can be transformative. Castor oil, rich in vitamin E and essential fatty acids, penetrates deeply to provide nourishment and hydration. Here's a simple, effective method to fortify your nails and moisturize your cuticles with castor oil:

Materials Needed:
- Pure, cold-pressed castor oil
- Cotton swabs or a small brush
- Gloves (optional for overnight treatment)

Step-by-Step Instructions:

1. Clean Your Nails: Start with clean, polish-free nails. Wash your hands with gentle soap and water, and dry them thoroughly.

2. Apply Castor Oil: Dip a cotton swab or a small brush into castor oil. Apply the oil directly onto each nail, ensuring full coverage from the nail bed to the tip. Don't forget to apply the oil to the underside of your nails if they are long enough.

3. Moisturize Cuticles: Using the same swab or brush, or even your fingertips, massage castor oil into your cuticles and the skin around your nails. This helps to soften the cuticles and prevent peeling or cracking.

4. Let It Absorb: Allow the oil to sit and deeply penetrate the nails and cuticles. For best results, do this treatment at night and consider wearing cotton gloves to bed. This not only helps the oil to stay in place but also keeps your hands warm, which can enhance absorption.

5. Repeat Nightly: Consistency is key for noticeable results. Apply castor oil to your nails and cuticles every night before bed. Within a few weeks, you should start to see stronger nails and healthier cuticles.

Additional Tips:
- Gentle Push Back Cuticles: After a week of nightly castor oil applications, your cuticles should be soft

enough to gently push back with a cuticle pusher. This should be done carefully to avoid damaging the nail bed.

- Avoid Harsh Chemicals: When cleaning or doing dishes, wear gloves to protect your nails from harsh detergents and chemicals that can strip moisture and weaken your nails.
- Hydration: Try to Keep your body well hydrated and drink plenty of water. Hydration is crucial for maintaining healthy nails and skin.
- Balanced Diet: Incorporate foods rich in biotin, protein, and omega-3 fatty acids into your diet to support nail health from the inside out.

By making castor oil a staple in your nail care routine, you can enjoy the benefits of stronger nails and softer cuticles. This simple, natural treatment not only enhances the appearance of your hands but also promotes overall nail health, preventing common issues like brittleness and splitting.

Castor Oil for Smoother, Hydrated Hands

For smoother, hydrated hands that feel soft to the touch and are visibly nourished, castor oil offers a natural, effective solution. Its rich composition deeply moisturizes the skin, addressing dryness and promoting a supple texture. Here's a step-by-step guide to creating a castor oil hand treatment that can be easily incorporated into your nightly routine.

Materials Needed:
- 2 tablespoons of castor oil
- 1 tablespoon of shea butter
- 1 teaspoon of aloe vera gel
- Small bowl for mixing
- Spoon or spatula for stirring
- Gloves (optional)

Instructions:

1. Prepare the Mixture: In a small bowl, combine the castor oil, shea butter, and aloe vera gel. Shea butter is known for its deep moisturizing properties, while aloe vera gel adds a soothing, cooling effect to the treatment.

2. Warm the Mixture: Gently warm the mixture to melt the shea butter and blend the ingredients thoroughly. This can be done in a microwave for a few seconds or over a double boiler. Ensure the mixture is comfortably warm, not hot, to maintain the therapeutic properties of the ingredients.

3. Apply to Your Hands: Once the mixture is warm and fully combined, use your fingers to apply it liberally to both hands. Pay special attention to dry areas, such as the knuckles and cuticles, massaging the mixture in circular motions to enhance absorption and stimulate blood flow.

4. Wear Gloves (Optional): For an intensive treatment, wear cotton gloves after applying the mixture. The gloves help to lock in moisture and warmth, increasing the efficacy of the treatment. Leave the gloves on for at least an hour, or overnight for best results.

5. Rinse Off: If you choose not to wear gloves, let the mixture absorb into your skin for 20-30 minutes, then rinse your hands with warm water. If you've worn gloves overnight, remove them in the morning and wash your hands as usual.

6. Repeat Regularly: For sustained softness and hydration, incorporate this castor oil hand treatment into your nightly routine. Regular use will result in smoother, more hydrated hands, with a noticeable improvement in skin texture and elasticity.

Additional Tips:
- Daily Maintenance: During the day, keep a small bottle of castor oil or a pre-made mixture of castor oil and your favorite hand cream at your desk or in your purse. A quick application can provide instant relief from dryness, especially in harsh weather conditions.
- Exfoliation: Once a week, exfoliate your hands with a gentle scrub to remove dead skin cells. This enhances the absorption of the castor oil treatment, making it even more effective.
- Sun Protection: Protect your hands from sun damage by applying a broad-spectrum sunscreen during the day. This prevents premature aging and maintains the health of your skin.

By following these steps, you can harness the moisturizing power of castor oil to achieve and maintain smooth, hydrated hands. This simple, natural treatment not only soothes and repairs dry skin but also promotes overall hand health, leaving your skin feeling soft and rejuvenated.

Book 4: Castor Oil for Lustrous Hair

Boosting Hair Growth and Thickness

The quest for thick, voluminous hair is common, yet achieving it can seem elusive. Castor oil, with its high content of ricinoleic acid, offers a natural pathway to not only boost hair growth but also improve hair thickness. This section delves into creating effective hair growth oil blends, incorporating scalp massages, and utilizing hot oil treatments to stimulate your scalp and encourage healthy hair growth.

Hair Growth Oil Blends: Castor Oil + Essential Oils

Combining castor oil with essential oils can create potent blends that target hair growth and scalp health. Here's how to make a basic hair growth oil blend:

Materials Needed:- 3 tablespoons of castor oil- 1 tablespoon of jojoba oil or coconut oil (as a carrier oil)- 5 drops of rosemary essential oil- 5 drops of peppermint essential oil- Dark glass bottle for storage

Instructions:

1. Mix Oils: In a bowl, combine the castor oil with your chosen carrier oil. These oils form the base of your blend, nourishing the scalp and hair.

2. Add Essential Oils: Stir in the rosemary and peppermint essential oils. Rosemary is known for promoting hair thickness and growth, while peppermint stimulates the scalp, encouraging hair growth.

3. Transfer to Bottle: Pour the blend into a dark glass bottle to protect the oils from light degradation.

4. Application: To use, apply a few drops to the scalp and massage gently. Focus on areas that need the most attention. Leave it on for at least 30 minutes or overnight for deeper penetration.

5. Rinse: Wash your hair with a gentle shampoo to remove the oil.

Scalp Massages and Hot Oil Treatments

Regular scalp massages increase blood flow to the hair follicles, which is essential for bringing nutrients to the hair roots and promoting growth. When combined with castor oil, this practice can significantly enhance hair health.

Hot Oil Treatment:- Warm a mixture of castor oil and a carrier oil in a heat-safe container. Test the temperature to ensure it's warm but not hot.- Apply the warm oil to your scalp and hair, massaging gently.- Cover your hair with a shower cap and wrap a warm towel around your head to increase absorption.-

Leave it on for at least 30 minutes before washing out with shampoo.

Treating Hair Loss, Thinning Hair, and Alopecia

Hair loss and thinning can be distressing, but castor oil's properties make it a valuable ally in treating these conditions. Its ability to reduce inflammation and support scalp health can help mitigate hair loss and encourage regrowth.

Routine for Addressing Hair Loss:- Apply a mixture of castor oil and a carrier oil directly to the scalp, focusing on areas of thinning.- Gently massage the scalp for several minutes to enhance blood circulation.- For best results, leave the treatment on overnight, covering your head with a breathable cap.- Wash your hair in the morning with a gentle, sulfate-free shampoo.

Maintaining Healthy, Shiny Hair

Beyond stimulating growth, castor oil is excellent for maintaining the overall health and shine of your hair. Its fatty acids can smooth the hair cuticle, adding a natural sheen and softness that enhances your hair's appearance.

Castor Oil Shampoos and Conditioners

Incorporating castor oil into your regular hair care routine can provide ongoing nourishment and protection. Look for shampoos and conditioners that contain castor oil as a key ingredient, or add a few drops of castor oil to your favorite products before use.

Hair Masks for Damage Repair and Shine

Create a weekly hair mask by mixing castor oil with ingredients like egg yolk, honey, or avocado. Apply the mask to damp hair, leave it on for 20-30 minutes, then rinse thoroughly. These treatments can deeply condition the hair, repair damage, and add a luminous shine.

Split Ends and Dry Scalp Treatments

Regular use of castor oil can help prevent split ends and soothe dry scalp conditions. Apply a small amount of oil to the ends of your hair to protect and moisturize. For dry scalp, massage castor oil directly onto the scalp before bed, and wash out in the morning.

Eyebrows, Eyelashes, and More

Castor oil's benefits extend beyond the scalp, promoting growth and thickness in eyebrows and eyelashes as well. Apply a small amount with a clean brush or cotton swab nightly for natural enhancement.

By integrating castor oil into your hair care regimen through these methods, you can achieve not only the growth and thickness you desire but also maintain the health and beauty of your hair.

Boosting Hair Growth and Thickness

Achieving thick, voluminous hair is a goal for many, and castor oil, rich in ricinoleic acid, is a natural ally in this quest. Its unique properties not only stimulate hair growth but also enhance hair thickness. Here's how to leverage castor oil for maximizing hair health and vitality.

Hair Growth Oil Blends: Castor Oil + Essential Oils

Creating a synergistic blend of castor oil with essential oils can amplify the benefits for hair growth and scalp health. Essential oils such as rosemary and peppermint are celebrated for their ability to invigorate the scalp and support hair growth, making them perfect companions to castor oil.- Materials Needed:- 3 tablespoons of castor oil- 1 tablespoon of jojoba oil or coconut oil (as a carrier oil)- 5 drops of rosemary essential oil- 5 drops of peppermint essential oil- Dark glass bottle for storage- Instructions:

1. Mix the castor oil with your chosen carrier oil in a bowl. This forms the nourishing base of your blend.

2. Stir in the rosemary and peppermint essential oils. These ingredients are key for stimulating the scalp and promoting hair growth.

3. Pour the blend into a dark glass bottle to preserve the integrity of the oils.

4. For application, massage a few drops into the scalp with gentle pressure. Focus on areas that are thinning or where you desire more growth. Leave it on for at least 30 minutes or overnight, then wash out with a gentle shampoo.

Scalp Massages and Hot Oil Treatments

Enhancing blood flow to the scalp is crucial for nourishing hair follicles and promoting healthy hair growth. Scalp massages, especially when performed with warm castor oil, can significantly boost circulation and effectiveness of the treatment.- Hot Oil Treatment Process:- Warm a mixture of castor oil and a carrier oil to a comfortable temperature.- Apply the warm oil to your scalp and through your hair, massaging gently to distribute the oil evenly.- Cover your hair with a shower cap and wrap a warm towel around your head to enhance absorption.- After at least 30 minutes, or for deeper penetration overnight, wash your hair with a gentle shampoo.

Addressing Hair Loss and Thinning Hair

Castor oil's anti-inflammatory and antimicrobial properties make it an effective solution for addressing scalp issues that contribute to hair loss and thinning hair. Regular application can create a healthier scalp environment conducive to hair regrowth.- Routine for Combatting Hair Loss:- Mix castor oil with a lighter carrier oil to facilitate easier application and absorption.- Apply this mixture to the scalp, focusing on areas of concern, and massage gently for several minutes.- Leave the treatment on overnight, covering your head with a breathable cap to avoid staining your linens.- In the morning, wash your hair with a sulfate-free shampoo to remove the oil without stripping the scalp of its natural oils.

Maintaining Healthy, Shiny Hair

Castor oil is not only beneficial for growth but also for the overall health of your hair. Its fatty acids can help to seal moisture in the hair shaft, reducing frizz and enhancing shine.- Incorporate Castor Oil into Your Regular Hair Care: Look for or create shampoos and conditioners that include castor oil as an ingredient. You can also add a few drops of castor oil to your existing hair care products for an extra moisture boost.- Weekly Hair Masks: Combine castor oil with natural ingredients like egg yolk, honey, or avocado for a nourishing hair mask. Apply to damp hair, leave on for 20-30 minutes, then rinse thoroughly. These treatments can help to repair damage, add shine, and improve hair texture.

By incorporating castor oil into your hair care regimen through these methods, you can support and enhance hair growth, combat thinning, and maintain the health and beauty of your hair. Regular use of castor oil, combined with essential oils and proper scalp care, can transform your hair, making it thicker, stronger, and more lustrous.

Hair Growth Oil Blends: Castor Oil + Essential Oils

Combining the potent properties of castor oil with the therapeutic benefits of essential oils creates a powerful synergy for stimulating hair growth and improving scalp health. This blend harnesses the nourishing power of castor oil, renowned for its ability to enhance hair thickness and growth, with the revitalizing effects of essential oils, each selected for their unique benefits to the scalp and hair follicles.

Materials Needed:- 3 tablespoons of castor oil- 1 tablespoon of grapeseed oil (as a carrier oil)- 5 drops of lavender essential oil- 5 drops of tea tree essential oil- Dark glass dropper bottle

Step-by-Step Instructions:

1. Prepare Your Blend: In a clean bowl, mix the castor oil with grapeseed oil. Grapeseed oil is chosen for its lightweight texture and ability to moisturize the scalp without leaving a greasy residue.

2. Add Essential Oils: Incorporate the lavender and tea tree essential oils into the oil mixture. Lavender essential oil is celebrated for its ability to promote hair growth, soothe the scalp, and improve

blood circulation. Tea tree oil contributes its antimicrobial properties, helping to unclog hair follicles and nourish the roots.

3. Transfer to Dropper Bottle: Carefully pour your oil blend into the dark glass dropper bottle. The dark glass helps preserve the integrity of the essential oils and castor oil by protecting them from light.

4. Application Method: To apply, section your hair and use the dropper to distribute the oil blend directly onto the scalp. Gently massage the oil into the scalp with your fingertips for several minutes to enhance absorption and stimulate blood flow. The massage itself is therapeutic and encourages hair growth by increasing circulation to the hair follicles.

5. Leave-In Treatment: For best results, allow the treatment to penetrate the scalp by leaving it on for at least an hour or overnight. If you choose to leave the oil in overnight, consider covering your pillow with a towel to protect your linens.

6. Washing Out: Rinse the oil blend from your hair using a gentle shampoo. It may require two washes to fully remove the oil, depending on your hair type. Follow up with your regular conditioner.

Frequency of Use: For optimal results, incorporate this hair growth oil blend into your hair care routine 2-3 times a week. Consistency is key to seeing significant improvements in hair growth and scalp health.

Additional Tips:- Always perform a patch test before using the blend extensively, especially if you have sensitive skin.- Adjust the essential oils based on your preferences or specific scalp needs. For instance, rosemary essential oil can be a great addition for its hair growth-promoting properties.- Stay patient and consistent. Hair growth takes time, and regular use of this blend can help achieve noticeable results over weeks to months.

This hair growth oil blend combines the best of nature's offerings to provide a natural, effective solution for those seeking to enhance their hair's growth and vitality. By nurturing the scalp and hair follicles with this potent mixture, you're setting the stage for healthier, thicker, and more lustrous hair.

Scalp Massages and Hot Oil Treatments

Scalp massages and hot oil treatments with castor oil are transformative practices that can significantly enhance hair health, promoting growth and thickness. These techniques stimulate the scalp, improving blood circulation, which is essential for nourishing the hair follicles and encouraging healthy hair growth. Here's how to incorporate these practices into your hair care routine for optimal results.

Materials Needed:- Pure, cold-pressed castor oil- A carrier oil (such as coconut or jojoba oil) to dilute the castor oil- A small bowl for mixing- A towel or shower cap- A microwave or hot water bath to warm the oil

Scalp Massage Instructions:

1. Prepare the Oil Blend: Mix 2 tablespoons of castor oil with 2 tablespoons of your chosen carrier oil in a small bowl. This dilution makes the thick castor oil easier to apply and massage into the scalp.

2. Warm the Oil: Gently warm the oil blend. You can do this by placing the bowl in a microwave for a few seconds or sitting it in a hot water bath. Ensure the oil is comfortably warm to touch, not hot, to avoid scalp burns.

3. Apply the Oil: Using your fingertips, apply the warm oil to your scalp. Start from the edges and work your way to the center, ensuring full coverage.

4. Massage: Use gentle, circular motions to massage the oil into your scalp for at least 5-10 minutes. Focus on areas that are prone to thinning to stimulate blood flow and encourage hair growth.

5. Cover and Wait: Once you've thoroughly massaged your scalp, cover your hair with a towel or shower cap. This traps the heat, enhancing the oil's penetration. Leave the oil on for at least 30 minutes, though overnight treatment is ideal for deeper conditioning.

6. Rinse: Wash your hair with a gentle shampoo to remove the oil. You may need to shampoo twice to ensure all oil is out, followed by your regular conditioner.

Hot Oil Treatment Instructions:

1. Prepare Your Oil: Mix equal parts castor oil and a carrier oil in a bowl. You'll need enough to cover your scalp and hair, depending on your hair length and thickness.

2. Warm the Oil: Warm the oil mixture as described above, checking the temperature to ensure it's safe for application.

3. Apply to Hair and Scalp: Work the warm oil through your hair from roots to ends, massaging into the scalp as you go.

4. Cover: Use a shower cap or towel to cover your hair. For added heat, you can warm a towel in the dryer and wrap it around your head.

5. Wait: Leave the oil in your hair for at least 30 minutes. For more intensive conditioning, you can leave it on overnight.

6. Wash Out: Rinse the oil from your hair with a gentle shampoo, following up with conditioner.

Benefits:- Enhanced Blood Circulation: Scalp massages increase blood flow to the hair follicles, delivering the nutrients necessary for hair growth.- Moisturization: Castor oil deeply moisturizes the scalp and hair, preventing dryness and promoting healthier hair growth.- Strength and Thickness: Regular treatments can strengthen hair, reduce breakage, and make hair appear thicker and fuller.

Incorporating scalp massages and hot oil treatments into your weekly hair care routine can lead to noticeable improvements in hair health and growth. With patience and consistency, these practices can help you achieve the lustrous, healthy hair you desire.

Treating Hair Loss, Thinning Hair, and Alopecia

Treating hair loss, thinning hair, and alopecia can be a challenging journey, but incorporating castor oil into your hair care regimen offers a natural and effective approach. Castor oil, renowned for its ricinoleic acid content, has been shown to improve scalp health, stimulate hair follicles, and promote hair growth. Here's a detailed guide on how to use castor oil to combat these concerns.

Materials Needed:- Pure, cold-pressed castor oil- Carrier oil (such as coconut, jojoba, or almond oil)- Shower cap or plastic wrap- Gentle shampoo and conditioner

Step-by-Step Instructions:

1. Prepare the Oil Mixture: Combine two tablespoons of castor oil with one tablespoon of your chosen carrier oil. This dilution makes the castor oil easier to apply and helps in spreading it evenly across the scalp.

2. Warm the Oil: Slightly warm the oil mixture to enhance its penetration into the scalp. Ensure it's comfortably warm to the touch, not hot, to avoid any scalp discomfort.

3. Apply to the Scalp: Using your fingertips or a cotton ball, apply the oil mixture directly onto the scalp, especially focusing on areas most affected by hair loss or thinning.

4. Massage Gently: Spend a few minutes massaging the oil into your scalp with gentle, circular motions. This not only helps in distributing the oil evenly but also stimulates blood circulation to the hair follicles.

5. Cover Your Head: Once the oil is applied, cover your hair with a shower cap or wrap your head with plastic wrap. This creates a warm environment that facilitates the oil's deeper penetration into the scalp.

6. Leave It On: For optimal results, leave the oil treatment on your scalp for at least an hour, though overnight treatment is highly recommended for maximum absorption.

7. Wash Your Hair: Rinse the oil from your hair using a gentle shampoo. It may require two washes to completely remove the oil. Follow up with a hydrating conditioner to keep your hair soft and manageable.

8. Repeat Regularly: Consistency is key in treating hair loss and thinning hair. Apply this treatment at least once a week to observe significant improvements over time.

Additional Tips:- Patch Test: Always perform a patch test before applying castor oil to your scalp, especially if you have sensitive skin, to ensure you don't have an allergic reaction.- Healthy Diet: Incorporate a diet rich in vitamins and minerals that support hair growth, such as Vitamin E, iron, and omega fatty acids, to complement the topical treatment with castor oil.- Stay Hydrated: Drinking adequate water daily helps in maintaining overall scalp health and supports hair growth.- Gentle Hair Care: Avoid tight hairstyles and harsh chemical treatments that can exacerbate hair loss and damage the hair follicles.- Stress Management: Since stress can be a contributing factor to hair loss, adopting stress-reduction techniques such as yoga, meditation, or regular exercise can be beneficial.

By following this comprehensive approach and incorporating castor oil into your hair care routine, you can effectively address hair loss, thinning hair, and alopecia. With patience and regular care, castor oil can help in restoring hair density and promoting a healthier, fuller head of hair.

Maintaining Healthy, Shiny Hair

For those seeking to maintain healthy, shiny hair, incorporating castor oil into your hair care routine can be a game-changer. Its unique properties not only promote hair growth but also enhance the natural sheen and strength of your locks. Here's how to leverage castor oil for lustrous, vibrant hair.

Deep Conditioning Treatments with Castor Oil

Deep conditioning treatments are essential for restoring moisture, improving elasticity, and adding shine to your hair. Castor oil, with its rich fatty acids, deeply penetrates the hair shaft, providing intense hydration and repair.- Materials Needed:- 2 tablespoons of castor oil- 1 tablespoon of coconut oil- Shower cap or warm towel- Instructions:

1. Mix the castor oil and coconut oil in a bowl. Coconut oil is added for its lightweight moisture and ability to help carry the thicker castor oil more deeply into the hair strands.

2. Warm the oil mixture slightly to enhance its penetration. Ensure it's comfortably warm to the touch.

3. Apply the warm oil blend to clean, damp hair, starting from the roots and working your way down

to the ends.

4. Once your hair is fully coated, cover it with a shower cap or wrap it in a warm towel to open up the hair cuticles and allow the oil to penetrate deeply.

5. Leave the treatment on for at least 30 minutes. For more intensive hydration, you can leave it on overnight.

6. Rinse your hair thoroughly with shampoo and follow up with conditioner.

Regular Scalp Massages

Scalp massages not only feel incredibly relaxing but also stimulate blood circulation, promoting healthy hair growth. When combined with castor oil, scalp massages nourish the roots and strengthen the hair.- Materials Needed:- A few drops of castor oil- Instructions:

1. Place a few drops of castor oil onto your fingertips.

2. Gently massage the oil into your scalp using circular motions. Focus on areas that feel tense or that are prone to dryness.

3. Continue the massage for about 5-10 minutes to ensure the oil is evenly distributed and the scalp is thoroughly stimulated.

4. For best results, leave the oil in your hair overnight and wash it out in the morning. If you're short on time, a 30-minute session before your shower is still beneficial.

Shiny Hair Rinse

A shiny hair rinse can help to seal the hair cuticles, locking in moisture and leaving your hair looking glossy and vibrant. This simple rinse can be used after your regular shampoo and conditioner routine.- Materials Needed:- 1 cup of cold water- 1 tablespoon of apple cider vinegar- 2-3 drops of castor oil- Instructions:

1. Combine the cold water, apple cider vinegar, and castor oil in a jug. Shake well to ensure the oil is somewhat dispersed in the mixture.

2. After conditioning, pour the rinse over your hair as a final step. The cold water helps to close the hair cuticles, while the apple cider vinegar clarifies the scalp and adds shine.

3. Do not rinse out. Allow your hair to air dry for maximum shine.

Protective Styling with Castor Oil

Protective styling minimizes hair manipulation, reducing breakage and moisture loss. Castor oil can be used to add an extra layer of protection and nourishment to your hair before styling.- Materials Needed:- A small amount of castor oil- Instructions:

1. Rub a small amount of castor oil between your palms.

2. Gently work the oil through your hair, focusing on the ends, which are the oldest and most prone to damage.

3. Style your hair as usual, whether it's braiding, twisting, or simply pulling it back into a protective style. The castor oil will help to keep your hair moisturized and protected throughout the day.

By incorporating these castor oil treatments into your hair care routine, you can maintain healthy, shiny hair that radiates vitality. Regular use of castor oil not only promotes growth but also enhances the natural beauty and strength of your hair, ensuring it remains lustrous and resilient against damage.

Castor Oil Shampoos and Conditioner

For those looking to enhance the health and appearance of their hair, integrating castor oil into your shampoo and conditioner routine offers a simple yet effective method. Castor oil, known for its rich fatty acids, particularly ricinoleic acid, provides deep nourishment to the scalp and hair follicles, promoting hair growth and restoring moisture to dry strands. Here's how to incorporate this powerful natural ingredient into your hair care regimen through shampoos and conditioners.

Creating Your Own Castor Oil Shampoo:

1. Choose a Mild Shampoo Base: Start with a gentle, sulfate-free shampoo as your base. This ensures that your hair and scalp are cleansed without stripping away natural oils.

2. Add Castor Oil: For every 8 ounces of shampoo, mix in 1 tablespoon of cold-pressed castor oil. This ratio can be adjusted based on your hair type; those with drier hair may benefit from a bit more oil, while those with oily hair should use less.

3. Incorporate Essential Oils (Optional): Enhance your shampoo with a few drops of essential oils such as peppermint or rosemary for additional scalp stimulation and hair growth benefits. About 5 drops per 8 ounces of shampoo is a good starting point.

4. Mix Thoroughly: Ensure the castor oil and optional essential oils are well integrated into the shampoo. Shake the bottle well before each use, as the oil may separate over time.

Formulating a Nourishing Castor Oil Conditioner:

1. Select a Hydrating Conditioner Base: Opt for a rich, moisturizing conditioner that aligns with your hair's hydration needs. A thicker, cream-based conditioner works well to lock in moisture.

2. Blend in Castor Oil: Add 1 tablespoon of castor oil to every 8 ounces of conditioner. This will not only amplify the conditioner's moisturizing properties but also leave your hair feeling soft and looking shiny.

3. Customize with Additional Oils (Optional): For extra conditioning, consider blending in other hair-friendly oils like coconut or argan oil, which can enhance softness and shine. A teaspoon of either oil will suffice.

4. Stir to Combine: Mix the oils into the conditioner thoroughly to ensure an even distribution. As with the shampoo, it's important to shake or stir the conditioner before use.

Application Tips:- Shampooing: When washing your hair, focus on massaging the castor oil-infused shampoo into the scalp to remove buildup and stimulate blood flow. This encourages healthy hair growth from the roots.- Conditioning: Apply the castor oil conditioner generously from mid-lengths to ends, avoiding the scalp to prevent greasiness. Leave it on for a few minutes to allow the hair to absorb the nutrients before rinsing thoroughly.- Frequency: Depending on your hair type, a castor oil shampoo and conditioner routine can be used 2-3 times a week. Pay attention to how your hair responds and adjust usage accordingly.

By customizing your shampoo and conditioner with castor oil, you're providing your hair with essential nutrients that promote growth, enhance shine, and improve overall hair health. This simple addition to your hair care routine can make a significant difference in the texture, appearance, and strength of your hair, helping you achieve the lustrous locks you desire.

Hair Masks for Damage Repair and Shine

Revitalize your hair with a deeply nourishing castor oil hair mask, designed to repair damage and restore a luminous shine. This treatment combines the powerful hydrating properties of castor oil with natural ingredients to create a potent remedy for dry, damaged hair. Follow these steps to concoct and apply a hair mask that not only mends but also enhances the natural beauty of your locks.

Materials Needed:- 2 tablespoons of castor oil- 1 tablespoon of honey- 1 ripe avocado- Shower cap

Instructions:

1. Prepare the Avocado: Begin by mashing the ripe avocado in a bowl until it reaches a smooth consistency. Avocado is rich in vitamins and fatty acids, making it an excellent ingredient for moisturizing and strengthening hair.

2. Mix Ingredients: Add the castor oil and honey to the mashed avocado. Honey acts as a humectant, drawing moisture into the hair, while castor oil penetrates the hair shaft to repair and protect.

3. Apply the Mask: Wet your hair slightly with warm water to open the hair cuticles. Apply the mask evenly throughout your hair, from roots to ends, focusing on damaged areas. Use a wide-tooth comb to ensure even distribution.

4. Cover Your Hair: Once the mask is applied, cover your hair with a shower cap. The cap traps heat, enhancing the mask's penetration and effectiveness.

5. Wait: Leave the mask on for at least 30 minutes. For deeper conditioning, you can extend this time up to an hour.

6. Rinse Thoroughly: Wash your hair with lukewarm water and a gentle shampoo to remove the mask. Follow up with a conditioner to seal in moisture.

7. Dry and Style: Pat your hair dry with a soft towel and style as usual. Avoid using high heat settings on hair dryers or styling tools immediately after treatment to prevent stress on your newly nourished hair.

Frequency of Use:

For best results, incorporate this hair mask into your beauty routine once a week. Regular use will gradually repair hair damage and enhance shine, leaving your hair healthier and more resilient.

Additional Tips:- For an extra boost of hydration, add a teaspoon of coconut oil to the mask. Coconut oil is known for its ability to deeply moisturize and add shine.- If you have oily hair, concentrate the application of the mask on the mid-lengths to ends of your hair, avoiding the scalp to prevent excess oiliness.- To maximize the benefits of the mask, wrap a warm towel around the shower cap. The added warmth will further open the hair cuticles and enhance the treatment's efficacy.

This castor oil hair mask is a powerful tool in your arsenal against hair damage. With its blend of natural ingredients, it offers a holistic approach to restoring hair health, repairing damage caused by styling, heat, and environmental stressors. Embrace this treatment as part of your journey towards achieving lustrous, vibrant, and healthy hair.

Split Ends and Dry Scalp Treatments

To combat split ends and alleviate dry scalp, incorporating castor oil into your hair care regimen offers a natural and effective solution. The rich nutrients and moisturizing properties of castor oil can help to repair damaged hair and soothe scalp dryness. Here's a guide to using castor oil for these common hair concerns.

For Split Ends:

Split ends occur when the hair shaft splits at the end, often due to heat styling, chemical treatments, or environmental damage. Castor oil can help to prevent and treat split ends by replenishing the hair's natural oils and improving its overall health.- Materials Needed:- Pure, cold-pressed castor oil- A small bowl- A soft hair brush or comb- Instructions:

1. Pour a small amount of castor oil into the bowl. You only need a few drops, as a little goes a long way.

2. Dip your fingertips into the oil, then gently apply it to the ends of your hair. Focus on the last inch or two where split ends are most common.

3. Use a soft brush or comb to evenly distribute the oil through the ends of your hair.

4. For best results, leave the oil on your hair for at least an hour or overnight. If you choose to leave it overnight, consider wrapping your hair or using a pillowcase you don't mind getting oily.

5. Wash your hair with a gentle shampoo to remove the oil, followed by your regular conditioner.

For Dry Scalp:

A dry scalp can be itchy, flaky, and uncomfortable. Castor oil's hydrating properties make it an excellent remedy for soothing and moisturizing the scalp.- Materials Needed:- Pure, cold-pressed castor oil- A small bowl- Shower cap or towel- Instructions:

1. Warm the castor oil in a small bowl. Test the oil with your fingertip to ensure it's a comfortable temperature for application.

2. Part your hair into sections and apply the warm oil directly to your scalp with your fingertips or a cotton ball.

3. Massage the oil into your scalp for several minutes. The massage not only helps with absorption but also increases blood circulation to the scalp.

4. Cover your hair with a shower cap or a warm towel to enhance the oil's penetration. Leave it on for at least 30 minutes, though overnight treatment is ideal for deep hydration.

5. Wash your hair with a gentle shampoo to remove the oil, ensuring to rinse thoroughly to prevent any residue.

Additional Tips:- Regular treatment with castor oil can significantly improve the health of your hair and scalp. Incorporate these treatments into your hair care routine once or twice a week for best results.- Always use cold-pressed, pure castor oil to ensure you're getting the most benefits without any added chemicals or preservatives.- For those with oily hair or scalp, concentrate the application of castor oil on the ends of your hair and avoid applying it directly to the scalp to prevent excess oiliness.

By following these steps, you can utilize castor oil to effectively treat split ends and dry scalp, promoting healthier, more resilient hair.

Eyebrows, Eyelashes, and More

Enhancing the appearance of eyebrows and eyelashes can significantly impact overall facial aesthetics, creating a more polished and youthful look. Castor oil, with its rich nutrients and fatty acids, is a natural remedy that promotes thicker, fuller brows and lashes. Here's how to incorporate castor oil into your beauty routine for optimal results.

Materials Needed:- Pure, cold-pressed castor oil- Clean mascara wand or cotton swab- Small container for storage

Eyebrow Growth Serum:

1. Prepare the Serum: Pour a small amount of castor oil into the container. If you have sensitive skin, you can dilute the castor oil with a carrier oil like almond or jojoba oil to minimize any potential irritation.

2. Application: Dip the clean mascara wand or cotton swab into the castor oil. Gently apply the oil to your eyebrows, focusing on sparse areas. Be careful not to apply too much pressure that might cause damage to the delicate skin.

3. Leave Overnight: For best results, apply the castor oil serum to your eyebrows before bedtime. This allows the oil ample time to penetrate and nourish the hair follicles.

4. Consistent Use: Repeat this process nightly. Consistency is key to seeing noticeable growth and thickness in your eyebrows.

Eyelash Thickening Treatment:

1. Clean Your Eyelashes: Ensure your eyelashes are clean and free of makeup. Using a gentle makeup remover can help prevent any potential clogging of the hair follicles.

2. Apply Castor Oil: Using a clean mascara wand or cotton swab, lightly coat your eyelashes with castor oil. Start from the base and move towards the tips, ensuring each lash is covered. Avoid getting the oil into your eyes.

3. Overnight Treatment: Leave the castor oil on your eyelashes overnight to maximize absorption and effectiveness.

4. Morning Cleanse: In the morning, gently wash your face and eyes to remove any residual oil.

Additional Tips for Eyebrows and Eyelashes:- Patch Test: Before applying castor oil to your eyebrows and eyelashes, conduct a patch test on a small area of skin to ensure you don't have an allergic reaction.- Avoid Overapplication: While it might be tempting to apply a large amount of castor oil, moderation is key. Overapplication can lead to clogged pores and irritation.- Patience and Persistence: Growth and thickening of eyebrows and eyelashes take time. Regular application over several weeks to months is necessary to achieve visible results.- Quality Matters: Always use high-quality, pure, cold-pressed castor oil to ensure the best results and minimize the risk of irritation.

By incorporating castor oil into your beauty regimen for eyebrows and eyelashes, you can naturally enhance their appearance, promoting growth and thickness. This simple, cost-effective method not only improves the look of your brows and lashes but also nourishes and conditions them, contributing to overall eye health and beauty.

Eyebrow Growth Serums and Treatments

Pouring a small amount of high-quality, pure, cold-pressed castor oil into a clean, small container marks the beginning of creating an effective eyebrow growth serum. This natural remedy, celebrated for its rich nutrients and fatty acids, is particularly potent in promoting thicker, fuller brows. For those with sensitive skin, consider diluting the castor oil with a carrier oil such as almond or jojoba oil to minimize any potential irritation.

Using a clean mascara wand or cotton swab, dip into the castor oil, gently applying the oil to your eyebrows, focusing on sparse areas. It's crucial to apply the oil with care, avoiding too much pressure that might cause damage to the delicate skin around the eyes.

For optimal results, it's recommended to apply the castor oil serum to your eyebrows before bedtime. This allows the oil ample time to penetrate and nourish the hair follicles, maximizing the growth potential. Consistency is key; thus, repeating this process nightly is essential for seeing noticeable growth and thickness in your eyebrows.

Materials Needed:- Pure, cold-pressed castor oil- Carrier oil (optional, for sensitive skin)- Clean mascara wand or cotton swab- Small container for storage

Instructions:

1. Prepare the Serum: If using, mix the castor oil with a carrier oil in your small container. This dilution can help those with sensitive skin.

2. Application: Dip the clean mascara wand or cotton swab into the castor oil. Apply gently across each eyebrow, targeting areas that are less dense.

3. Overnight Treatment: Leave the serum on your eyebrows overnight to allow the oil to deeply condition and stimulate growth.

4. Consistent Use: Apply the serum nightly. Regular, uninterrupted application is crucial for achieving and maintaining results.

Additional Tips for Eyebrows and Eyelashes:- Conduct a patch test on a small area of skin before applying castor oil to your eyebrows to ensure you don't have an allergic reaction.- Use moderation in application; a small amount of oil is sufficient. Overapplication can lead to clogged pores and irritation.- Be patient and persistent. Eyebrow growth takes time, and regular application over several weeks to months is necessary for visible results.- Always opt for high-quality, pure, cold-pressed castor oil to ensure the best results and minimize the risk of irritation.

By incorporating castor oil into your beauty regimen for eyebrows and eyelashes, you can naturally enhance their appearance, promoting growth and thickness. This simple, cost-effective method not only improves the look of your brows and lashes but also nourishes and conditions them, contributing to overall eye health and beauty.

Conditioning and Lengthening Eyelash Serums

For those seeking to enhance the natural beauty of their eyelashes, incorporating a conditioning and lengthening serum made with castor oil can be a game-changer. This simple yet effective treatment leverages the nourishing properties of castor oil to promote healthier, longer, and more luscious lashes. Here's how to create and apply your own eyelash serum at home.

Materials Needed:- Pure, cold-pressed castor oil- Empty, clean mascara tube or small glass dropper bottle- Clean mascara wand or eyeliner brush

Instructions:

1. Fill the Container: Carefully pour castor oil into the empty mascara tube or glass dropper bottle. If using a dropper bottle, ensure it's equipped with a small enough dropper for precise application.

2. Application: In the evening, after removing all makeup and cleansing your face, apply a small amount of the castor oil serum to the base of your upper and lower eyelashes. Use the clean mascara wand or an eyeliner brush for a more precise application, ensuring minimal oil gets into the eyes.

3. Gentle Massage: Optionally, you can gently massage the eyelid area and lash line with your fingertips to further stimulate circulation and encourage growth. Be careful not to press too hard or get the oil directly into your eyes.

4. Leave Overnight: Allow the castor oil serum to work its magic overnight. This gives ample time for the oil to deeply penetrate the hair follicles, maximizing nourishment and growth potential.

5. Morning Routine: In the morning, gently wash your face and eye area to remove any residual oil. Proceed with your regular skincare and makeup routine.

Frequency of Use:

For best results, incorporate this eyelash serum into your nightly routine. Consistent use is key to achieving noticeable improvements in lash length, thickness, and overall health.

Additional Tips:- Always use high-quality, pure, cold-pressed castor oil to ensure the safety and effectiveness of your eyelash serum.- If you experience any irritation or discomfort, discontinue use immediately and consult with a healthcare professional.- Patience is crucial, as natural lash growth can take several weeks to become noticeable. Keep a consistent application schedule for at least 2-3 months to properly evaluate the benefits.- To maintain the hygiene of your serum, regularly clean the applicator wand or brush and avoid sharing your serum with others.

By following these steps, you can harness the power of castor oil to create a natural, conditioning, and lengthening eyelash serum. This easy-to-make beauty treatment not only promotes the growth of stronger, healthier lashes but also adds an extra layer of care to your nightly beauty regimen, helping you achieve the beautiful, fluttery eyelashes you desire.

Tips for Fuller and Defined Brows

Achieving fuller and more defined brows can significantly enhance your facial features and overall appearance. Castor oil, known for its rich nutrients and fatty acids, is a natural remedy that promotes hair growth and thickness. Here's how to use castor oil effectively for your eyebrows.

Materials Needed:- Pure, cold-pressed castor oil- Fine-tipped brush or clean mascara wand- Small container for castor oil

Step-by-Step Guide:

1. Cleanse Your Eyebrows: Start with a clean base by gently washing your face and eyebrows. Removing dirt and makeup ensures the castor oil can penetrate the hair follicles without obstruction.

2. Prepare the Castor Oil: Pour a small amount of castor oil into a small container. If you have sensitive skin, consider mixing the castor oil with a carrier oil like almond or jojoba to dilute its potency and minimize the risk of irritation.

3. Apply with Precision: Dip your fine-tipped brush or clean mascara wand into the castor oil. Wipe off any excess oil to avoid overapplication. Carefully apply the oil along your eyebrows, focusing on sparse areas. The key is to coat each hair lightly without saturating the skin underneath.

4. Massage Gently: Using your fingertips, softly massage the oil into your eyebrows for a minute or two. This helps stimulate blood circulation to the area, encouraging hair growth and allowing the oil to penetrate deeper into the follicles.

5. Leave Overnight: For best results, leave the castor oil on your eyebrows overnight. This gives the oil ample time to work, nourishing and strengthening the hair follicles for thicker growth.

6. Rinse in the Morning: Wash your face and eyebrows with your regular cleanser in the morning to remove the castor oil. Follow up with your usual skincare routine.

Frequency of Application:

For noticeable results, apply castor oil to your eyebrows every night. Consistency is crucial, as hair growth varies from person to person. Give it at least a few weeks to see improvements.

Additional Tips:- Patch Test: Always perform a patch test before applying castor oil to your eyebrows, especially if you have sensitive skin.- Be Patient: Eyebrow growth takes time. Regular, consistent application is essential for seeing the benefits of castor oil.- Avoid Over-Plucking: While you're using castor oil to encourage growth, try to minimize plucking or waxing. Over-grooming can hinder your progress towards fuller brows.- Healthy Diet: Incorporating a diet rich in vitamins and minerals can support hair growth from the inside out. Foods high in omega-3 fatty acids, biotin, and vitamins E and D are particularly beneficial.

By following these steps, you can utilize castor oil as a natural, effective way to achieve fuller and more defined eyebrows. With patience and consistent care, you'll be able to enhance the natural beauty of your brows, framing your face more prominently and boosting your confidence.

Book 5: Castor Oil for Anti-Aging and Timeless Beauty

Preventing Premature Aging

The natural aging process is inevitable, but premature aging can be combated with the right skincare routine. Castor oil, rich in antioxidants and fatty acids, offers a natural solution to protect the skin from environmental stressors that accelerate aging. Here's how to create a collagen-boosting face serum using castor oil to enhance skin elasticity and reduce the appearance of fine lines and wrinkles.

Collagen-Boosting Face Serum

Materials Needed:- 2 tablespoons of castor oil- 1 tablespoon of rosehip oil- 1 tablespoon of vitamin E oil- 5 drops of geranium essential oil- Dark glass dropper bottle

Instructions:

1. Combine Oils: In a small bowl, mix the castor oil, rosehip oil, and vitamin E oil. These oils work together to hydrate the skin, promote collagen production, and provide antioxidant protection.

2. Add Essential Oil: Incorporate the geranium essential oil into the mixture. Geranium is known for its ability to tighten skin, reduce wrinkles, and improve skin tone.

3. Transfer to Dropper Bottle: Carefully pour the serum into the dark glass dropper bottle to preserve the oils' integrity.

4. Application: Each night, after cleansing your face, apply 2-3 drops of the serum to your face and neck. Gently massage in upward motions until fully absorbed.

5. Storage: Try to keep the serum in a cool and dark place to maintain its potency.

Skin Tightening and Firming Solutions

Sagging skin and loss of firmness are common signs of aging that can be addressed with targeted treatments. Castor oil's fatty acids deeply moisturize the skin, improving its firmness and texture. Here's a method for creating a neck and décolletage firming oil.

Neck and Décolletage Firming Oils

Materials Needed:- 3 tablespoons of castor oil- 2 tablespoons of jojoba oil- 5 drops of frankincense essential oil- 5 drops of lavender essential oil- Small glass bottle

Instructions:

1. Prepare the Blend: Mix the castor oil and jojoba oil in a bowl. Jojoba oil is added for its similarity to the skin's natural oils, enhancing absorption.

2. Add Essential Oils: Stir in the frankincense and lavender essential oils. Frankincense is beneficial for its skin regeneration properties, while lavender soothes and heals the skin.

3. Bottle the Oil: Pour the mixture into the glass bottle for easy application.

4. Use: Massage a few drops of the oil onto your neck and décolletage area in upward strokes each night before bed.

5. Consistency: For best results, use consistently as part of your nightly skincare routine.

Overall Wellness and Longevity

Castor oil's benefits extend beyond topical applications; it can also support overall wellness, which in turn contributes to a youthful appearance. Here's how to incorporate castor oil into a detoxification routine to promote internal health and vitality.

Detoxification and Lymphatic Drainage

Materials Needed:- Cold-pressed castor oil- Wool flannel or cotton cloth- Plastic wrap- Hot water bottle or heating pad- Old towel

Instructions:

1. Prepare the Area: Choose a comfortable, quiet space where you can lie down for at least 30 minutes.

2. Apply Castor Oil: Soak the wool flannel or cotton cloth in castor oil and place it over your abdomen.

3. Cover: Wrap the plastic wrap around your abdomen to hold the cloth in place.

4. Apply Heat: Place the hot water bottle or heating pad over the wrapped area to enhance the oil's penetration and stimulate the lymphatic system.

5. Rest: Lie down and relax for 30-60 minutes. This is an excellent time for meditation or deep breathing exercises.

6. Clean Up: After removing the pack, cleanse the area with a mixture of baking soda and water to remove any residual oil.

Incorporating these castor oil-based treatments into your beauty and wellness routine can significantly contribute to anti-aging efforts, promoting not only timeless beauty but also overall health and vitality.

Preventing Premature Aging

Harnessing the power of castor oil for preventing premature aging taps into its rich content of antioxidants, essential fatty acids, and vitamin E, which collectively fortify the skin's barrier, enhance elasticity, and smooth fine lines. This natural approach not only addresses the visible signs of aging but also nourishes the skin at a cellular level, promoting a youthful, radiant complexion over time.

Collagen-Boosting Face Serum with Castor Oil

Creating a daily serum that leverages castor oil's ability to stimulate collagen production is a proactive step towards maintaining firm, youthful skin. Collagen, the protein responsible for skin elasticity, diminishes with age, but with the right nourishment, its degradation can be slowed.

Materials Needed:- 2 tablespoons of castor oil- 1 tablespoon of rosehip oil- 1 tablespoon of vitamin E oil- 5 drops of geranium essential oil- Dark glass dropper bottle

Instructions:

1. In a clean bowl, blend the castor oil, rosehip oil, and vitamin E oil. This combination offers a potent mix of antioxidants and fatty acids essential for skin repair and hydration.

2. Add the geranium essential oil to the mix. Known for its astringent properties, geranium oil helps tighten the skin, reducing the appearance of wrinkles.

3. Transfer the serum to the dark glass dropper bottle. The dark glass helps preserve the efficacy of the oils by protecting them from light degradation.

4. To apply, dispense 2-3 drops of the serum onto your fingertips and gently massage into clean, damp skin each night. Focus on areas prone to wrinkles, such as around the eyes, forehead, and mouth.

5. Store the serum in a cool, dark place to maintain its potency.

Hydrating Castor Oil Night Cream

A deeply moisturizing night cream enriched with castor oil can provide intense hydration, essential for repairing the skin overnight. Dry skin accelerates the appearance of aging, making hydration a key factor in a preventative skincare routine.

Materials Needed:- ¼ cup of shea butter- 1 tablespoon of castor oil- 1 tablespoon of jojoba oil- 5 drops of lavender essential oil- Small jar or container

Instructions:

1. Melt the shea butter using a double boiler method until it's just liquid. Shea butter offers a rich base that deeply moisturizes and repairs skin.

2. Remove from heat and stir in the castor oil and jojoba oil. These oils are excellent for their hydrating and healing properties, making them ideal for mature or dry skin types.

3. Once slightly cooled, add the lavender essential oil for its soothing and anti-inflammatory benefits.

4. Pour the mixture into your jar or container and let it solidify. If in a hurry, you can place it in the refrigerator.

5. Use this cream as the last step in your nighttime skincare routine, applying a small amount to your face and neck after the serum has absorbed.

Revitalizing Eye Treatment

The delicate skin around the eyes is often the first to show signs of aging. A targeted eye treatment using castor oil can help reduce the appearance of fine lines and dark circles.

Materials Needed:- 1 tablespoon of castor oil- 1 tablespoon of almond oil- Small roller bottle

Instructions:

1. Combine the castor oil and almond oil in the roller bottle. Almond oil is light and penetrates easily, making it perfect for the sensitive area around the eyes.

2. Shake well to mix.

3. Each night, after applying your serum and night cream, gently roll the oil blend around the eyes, focusing on the under-eye area and crow's feet.

4. Use your ring finger to lightly tap the oil into the skin, promoting absorption and stimulating circulation.

Incorporating these castor oil-based treatments into your daily skincare routine can significantly contribute to preventing premature aging. By nourishing the skin with essential nutrients, promoting hydration, and protecting against environmental damage, you can maintain a youthful, vibrant complexion for years to come.

Collagen-Boosting Face Serum

Harness the rejuvenating power of castor oil with this collagen-boosting face serum, designed to enhance skin elasticity and diminish the appearance of fine lines. Rich in ricinoleic acid, castor oil penetrates deep into the skin, promoting the production of collagen and elastin, essential proteins that keep your skin firm and youthful. Blended with complementary oils, this serum offers a potent mix that nourishes, hydrates, and revitalizes the skin.

Materials Needed:- 2 tablespoons of castor oil- 1 tablespoon of rosehip oil- 1 tablespoon of vitamin E oil- 5 drops of lavender essential oil- Dark glass dropper bottle

Step-by-Step Instructions:

1. Blend the Oils: In a clean mixing bowl, combine the castor oil, rosehip oil, and vitamin E oil. Rosehip oil is renowned for its skin-regenerating properties and high antioxidant content, while vitamin E provides additional nourishment and protection against environmental damage.

2. Incorporate Lavender Oil: Add the lavender essential oil to your blend. Lavender not only soothes the skin but also adds a calming, therapeutic fragrance to your serum.

3. Transfer to Dropper Bottle: Carefully pour your serum into the dark glass dropper bottle. The dark glass helps protect the oils from light, preserving their therapeutic properties.

4. Application: Each evening, after cleansing your face, apply 2-3 drops of the serum to your fingertips. Gently massage into your face and neck with upward motions, focusing on areas prone to wrinkles. The serum's lightweight formula allows for quick absorption, leaving your skin feeling soft and hydrated without a greasy residue.

5. Storage: Keep your collagen-boosting serum in a cool, dark place to maintain its efficacy. Avoid exposure to direct sunlight or extreme temperatures.

Benefits:- Enhanced Collagen Production: Regular use of the serum stimulates collagen production, improving skin elasticity and reducing the appearance of fine lines and wrinkles.- Deep Hydration: The combination of oils deeply moisturizes the skin, locking in hydration and leaving your complexion radiant and plump.- Antioxidant Protection: Rich in antioxidants, this serum helps to protect the skin from oxidative stress and environmental pollutants, preventing premature aging.- Soothing and Healing: Lavender essential oil not only adds a relaxing scent but also has properties that soothe and heal the skin, making this serum ideal for nighttime rejuvenation.

For best results, incorporate this collagen-boosting face serum into your nightly skincare routine. With consistent use, you'll notice a significant improvement in your skin's texture, firmness, and overall appearance, revealing a more youthful, radiant complexion.

Eye Creams for Puffiness and Dark Circles

Dark circles and puffiness under the eyes are common concerns that can make you look tired and older than you feel. Fortunately, castor oil, with its anti-inflammatory and moisturizing properties, offers a natural solution to these issues. Creating an eye cream with castor oil not only helps reduce puffiness and dark circles but also nourishes the delicate skin around the eyes, promoting a more youthful and refreshed appearance.

Materials Needed:- 1 tablespoon of castor oil- 1 tablespoon of aloe vera gel- ½ teaspoon of beeswax- 5 drops of chamomile essential oil- Small glass jar

Instructions:

1. Melt the Beeswax: In a double boiler, gently melt the beeswax. Beeswax forms the base of your cream, providing a protective barrier that locks in moisture and nourishment.

2. Combine Castor Oil and Aloe Vera: Once the beeswax has melted, remove it from the heat and stir in the castor oil and aloe vera gel. Aloe vera gel adds a soothing and cooling effect, perfect for reducing puffiness, while castor oil deeply moisturizes and targets dark circles.

3. Add Chamomile Essential Oil: Stir in the chamomile essential oil. Chamomile is known for its calming properties, which can help soothe the skin and reduce inflammation, making it ideal for treating the under-eye area.

4. Transfer to Glass Jar: Carefully pour the mixture into a small glass jar. Allow it to cool and solidify. The consistency should be creamy and easy to apply.

5. Application: Use your ring finger to gently apply a small amount of the cream to the under-eye area. The ring finger naturally applies less pressure, making it perfect for the delicate skin around the eyes. Apply in the evening before bed and in the morning as needed, allowing the cream to absorb fully.

Storage: Keep the eye cream in a cool and dark place. The shelf life should be several months, but if you notice any change in texture or smell, it's time to make a fresh batch.

Benefits:- Reduction in Puffiness and Dark Circles: Regular use of this eye cream can significantly reduce the appearance of puffiness and dark circles, thanks to the anti-inflammatory properties of castor oil and chamomile.

- Moisturizing: Castor oil deeply hydrates the skin, improving elasticity and reducing the appearance of fine lines and wrinkles around the eyes.- Soothing: Aloe vera and chamomile provide a soothing effect, reducing irritation and calming the skin.

This homemade eye cream is a gentle, effective way to address under-eye puffiness and dark circles. Incorporating it into your daily skincare routine can help you achieve a more youthful, awake appearance, naturally.

Night Oils for Deep Moisturization

For those seeking an intensive hydration treatment that works while you sleep, creating a night oil blend with castor oil can deeply moisturize and rejuvenate your skin. Castor oil, known for its thick and enriching properties, acts as a powerful emollient to lock in moisture, making it an ideal ingredient for a night-time facial oil. This blend also incorporates other natural oils to enhance the moisturizing effects and provide a soothing, aromatic experience that promotes relaxation before bed.

Materials Needed:- 2 tablespoons of castor oil- 1 tablespoon of jojoba oil- 1 tablespoon of sweet almond oil- 5 drops of lavender essential oil- Dark glass bottle with dropper

Instructions:

1. Mix the Oils: In a small bowl, combine the castor oil, jojoba oil, and sweet almond oil. Jojoba oil is closely matched to the skin's natural sebum, making it an excellent carrier for deep moisturization, while sweet almond oil is rich in vitamin E and keeps your skin cells healthy.

2. Add Lavender Essential Oil: Incorporate the lavender essential oil into your oil blend. Lavender not only has a calming scent that prepares you for a restful sleep but also possesses properties that can soothe and heal the skin overnight.

3. Bottle Your Blend: Transfer the completed blend into your dark glass bottle using a small funnel if necessary. The dark glass helps to preserve the integrity of the oils by protecting them from light degradation.

4. Application: Before bedtime, after you've cleansed your face and applied any water-based treatments or serums, dispense 2-3 drops of the night oil into the palm of your hand. Rub your hands together to warm the oil slightly, then gently press and massage the oil into your face and neck. Focus on areas that are particularly dry or where you want to enhance skin elasticity and reduce the appearance of fine lines.

5. Storage: Keep your night oil in a cool, dark place to maintain its potency. Ensure the cap is tightly sealed after each use to keep the essential oil fragrance intact.

Benefits:- Deep Hydration: This night oil blend provides an intense level of hydration, penetrating deeply into the skin to restore moisture lost during the day.- Skin Repair: The overnight hours are prime time for skin repair, and this oil blend supports the skin's natural regeneration process, helping to reduce the appearance of fine lines and wrinkles.- Soothing Aroma: The addition of lavender essential oil helps to relax the mind and body, promoting a more restful sleep which is crucial for skin health.

Frequency of Use:

For best results, incorporate this night oil into your daily evening skincare routine. Regular use will result in softer, more hydrated skin, with an improved texture and a radiant glow.

By dedicating a few minutes each night to applying this deeply moisturizing oil, you're not only giving your skin the nourishment it needs to repair and rejuvenate but also creating a moment of self-care that calms and prepares you for a restful night's sleep.

Skin Tightening and Firming Solutions

For those seeking natural methods to maintain and enhance skin elasticity, castor oil emerges as a potent ally. Its unique composition, rich in ricinoleic acid, not only deeply moisturizes but also tightens the skin, offering a non-invasive solution to achieving a firmer, more youthful complexion. Here, we explore innovative ways to incorporate castor oil into your skincare regimen for skin tightening and firming benefits.

Castor Oil and Egg White Mask for Facial Firming

Egg whites are renowned for their skin-tightening effects, which, when combined with the hydrating properties of castor oil, create a powerful facial mask for enhancing skin firmness.- Materials Needed:- 1 tablespoon of castor oil- 1 egg white- Mixing bowl- Whisk or fork- Brush for application- Instructions:

1. In your mixing bowl, whisk the egg white until frothy. Egg whites help tighten pores and lift the skin.

2. Add the castor oil to the whisked egg white, blending thoroughly to form a cohesive mixture.

3. Use the brush to apply the mask evenly across your face, avoiding the eye area.

4. Allow the mask to sit for 15-20 minutes or until it feels tight and has dried.

5. Rinse off with lukewarm water, patting your face dry with a soft towel.

Castor Oil Massage for Neck and Jawline

A regular massage with castor oil can stimulate blood circulation, enhancing skin elasticity and firmness, particularly around the neck and jawline where skin sagging often occurs.- Materials Needed:- 2 tablespoons of castor oil- Warm towel- Instructions:

1. Warm the castor oil slightly in a microwave-safe container for a few seconds until it is comfortably warm.

2. Apply the warm oil to your neck and jawline using upward strokes.

3. Gently massage the areas with your fingertips in circular motions for 5-10 minutes to boost blood flow and encourage tightening.

4. Soak the towel in hot water, wring out the excess, and place it over the treated areas until it cools to room temperature. The warmth helps open pores, allowing the castor oil to penetrate deeply.

5. Repeat this massage routine 2-3 times a week for optimal results.

Almond and Castor Oil Blend for Body Firming

Combining almond oil with castor oil enhances the skin's texture and firmness, making this blend ideal for body application, especially on areas prone to sagging like the stomach, arms, and thighs.- Materials Needed:- ¼ cup of castor oil- ¼ cup of almond oil- Glass bottle for storage- Instructions:

1. Mix equal parts of castor oil and almond oil in the glass bottle. Shake well to combine.

2. After showering, while your skin is still damp, apply the oil blend to your body, focusing on areas that need firming.

3. Massage the oil into your skin with firm, circular motions until fully absorbed.

4. For enhanced absorption and benefits, consider using a body brush to exfoliate your skin before applying the oil blend.

Hydration and Nutrition for Skin Firmness

While topical applications of castor oil provide direct benefits, maintaining skin firmness also requires adequate hydration and nutrition.- Hydration: Drink plenty of water throughout the day to keep your skin hydrated from the inside out. Proper hydration is crucial for maintaining skin elasticity.- Nutrition:

Incorporate foods rich in antioxidants, vitamins A, C, and E, and omega-3 fatty acids into your diet. These nutrients support skin health, promoting firmness and preventing premature aging.

By integrating these castor oil-based treatments into your skincare routine, you can naturally enhance skin firmness and elasticity. Regular use, combined with a healthy lifestyle, will contribute to a visibly tighter, more youthful complexion.

Neck and Décolletage Firming Oils

Creating a neck and décolletage firming oil blend with castor oil is a natural and effective way to address the signs of aging in these often-neglected areas. The skin on the neck and décolletage is thinner and more prone to dryness, making it more susceptible to sagging and wrinkles. Castor oil, known for its deep moisturizing properties and ability to promote skin elasticity, serves as the perfect base for a firming oil blend. Here's how to create and use your own neck and décolletage firming oil for a smoother, more youthful appearance.

Materials Needed:- 3 tablespoons of castor oil- 2 tablespoons of pomegranate seed oil- 5 drops of frankincense essential oil- 5 drops of rosehip essential oil- Small glass bottle with dropper

Instructions:

1. Prepare the Blend: In a small bowl, combine the castor oil with pomegranate seed oil. Pomegranate seed oil is rich in antioxidants and promotes skin regeneration, complementing the hydrating effects of castor oil.

2. Add Essential Oils: Stir in the frankincense and rosehip essential oils. Frankincense is known for its ability to reduce the appearance of fine lines and improve skin tone, while rosehip essential oil aids in skin repair and renewal.

3. Bottle the Oil: Carefully pour the mixture into the glass bottle. The dropper will make application easier and more precise.

4. Use: To apply, cleanse the neck and décolletage area and pat dry. Then, place a few drops of the oil blend onto your palms, rub them together to warm the oil slightly, and gently massage onto the neck and décolletage in upward strokes. Focus on areas that show signs of sagging or wrinkles.

5. Frequency: For best results, use the firming oil blend each night before bed. This allows the oils to work in tandem with the skin's natural repair processes that occur during sleep.

Additional Tips:- Consistency is Key: Regular use is essential for seeing noticeable results. Incorporate this firming oil into your nightly skincare routine for at least a few months to observe improvements in skin firmness and texture.- Gentle Massage: Use gentle, upward motions to massage the oil into the skin. This not only helps with absorption but also stimulates blood flow, which is beneficial for skin health and elasticity.- Sun Protection: The neck and décolletage area are exposed to the sun just as much as the face, so don't forget to apply sunscreen during the day to protect against UV damage, which can accelerate skin aging.

By dedicating a few minutes each night to applying this nourishing and firming oil blend, you can help maintain the skin's elasticity, reduce the appearance of wrinkles, and promote a more youthful look for your neck and décolletage.

Cellulite Reduction and Skin Smoothing Treatments

Cellulite, a common concern for many, appears as dimpled, uneven skin primarily on the thighs, hips, buttocks, and abdomen. It results from fat pushing through the connective tissue beneath the skin. While completely eliminating cellulite is challenging, certain treatments can reduce its appearance and smooth the skin. Castor oil, with its ricinoleic acid content, promotes the breakdown of fats and improves lymphatic drainage, making it an effective natural remedy for cellulite reduction.

Materials Needed:- Pure, cold-pressed castor oil- Dry brush or exfoliating glove- Glass bottle with dropper- Essential oils (optional): grapefruit, lemon, or rosemary for added benefits

Instructions:

1. Prepare Your Skin: Begin with dry brushing or using an exfoliating glove on dry skin before showering. This process exfoliates dead skin cells, boosts circulation, and enhances lymphatic drainage, preparing the skin to absorb the castor oil more effectively.

2. Mix the Treatment Oil: In a glass bottle, mix 3 tablespoons of castor oil with 5 drops of your chosen essential oil. Grapefruit, lemon, and rosemary essential oils are known for their ability to improve blood circulation and promote the breakdown of fat deposits under the skin.

3. Warm the Oil: Slightly warm the oil mixture by placing the glass bottle in a bowl of hot water for a few minutes. Test the oil on your wrist to ensure it's a comfortable temperature.

4. Apply the Oil: After showering and patting your skin dry, apply the warm oil to areas affected by cellulite. Massage the oil into your skin using firm, circular motions. For enhanced penetration, use a massage brush or your hands to vigorously massage the oil, focusing on problematic areas.

5. Wrap the Area (Optional): For a more intensive treatment, after applying the oil, wrap the area with plastic wrap and cover with a warm towel for 20-30 minutes. This "castor oil pack" method allows deeper penetration of the oil and a more pronounced detoxifying effect.

6. Rinse Off: If you choose to wrap the area, remove the plastic wrap after the specified time and take a warm shower to rinse off any residual oil.

7. Repeat Regularly: For best results, perform this treatment 2-3 times a week. Consistency is key to seeing a reduction in cellulite and an improvement in skin texture.

Additional Tips:- Stay Hydrated: Drinking plenty of water helps flush toxins from the body, complementing the detoxifying effects of the castor oil treatment.- Maintain a Healthy Diet: A diet rich in fruits, vegetables, and lean proteins can support skin health and reduce the appearance of cellulite.- Exercise Regularly: Engaging in regular physical activity, especially exercises that target areas prone to cellulite, can help tone the body and reduce fat deposits.

By incorporating this castor oil treatment into your skincare routine, you can naturally reduce the appearance of cellulite and achieve smoother, more toned skin. Remember, while castor oil can significantly improve skin texture and appearance, a holistic approach including diet, hydration, and exercise will yield the best results.

Castor Oil Body Wraps for Toning

Castor oil body wraps are a luxurious, spa-like treatment you can do at home to help tone and tighten your skin. This method leverages the potent anti-inflammatory and moisturizing properties of castor oil, combined with the heat and pressure of the wrap, to detoxify and improve skin elasticity. Here's how to create your own castor oil body wrap for an at-home toning experience.

Materials Needed:- Pure, cold-pressed castor oil- Plastic wrap- Warm towel or heating pad- Cotton or wool cloth large enough to cover the targeted area- Comfortable, warm space where you can relax for at least 30 minutes

Step-by-Step Instructions:

1. Prepare the Skin: Start with clean, dry skin. Gently exfoliate the area you plan to treat to remove dead skin cells and enhance the oil's absorption.

2. Warm the Castor Oil: Warm a sufficient amount of castor oil so it feels comfortable on the skin. You can do this by placing the oil in a glass container and then placing the container in warm water. Do not microwave the oil as this can destroy its beneficial properties.

3. Apply Castor Oil: Soak the cotton or wool cloth in the warm castor oil. Wring out the excess oil so the cloth is saturated but not dripping. Apply the cloth to the area you wish to tone, such as the abdomen, thighs, or arms.

4. Wrap the Area: Carefully wrap the plastic wrap around the cloth-covered area. The plastic wrap helps maintain the warmth and ensures the cloth stays in place. Avoid wrapping too tightly; the goal is to feel comfortable and allow your skin to breathe.

5. Add Heat: Place a warm towel or heating pad over the plastic wrap. This step helps open the pores, allowing the castor oil to penetrate deeply into the skin. The heat also enhances circulation and aids in the detoxification process.

6. Relax: Lie down in a comfortable, warm space and relax for at least 30 minutes. This is a great time to meditate, listen to soothing music, or simply rest. The warmth, combined with the castor oil's properties, works to detoxify and tone your skin.

7. Remove and Cleanse: After 30 minutes, remove the plastic wrap and wash the treated area with warm water. You can use a mild soap if desired. Pat the skin dry with a clean towel.

8. Hydrate: Follow up with a light moisturizer or aloe vera gel to hydrate the skin and enhance the toning effects of the wrap.

Frequency of Use:

For best results, use the castor oil body wrap once a week. Consistent use, combined with a healthy diet and regular exercise, can lead to visibly toned and tightened skin over time.

Benefits:- Detoxifies the body by promoting lymphatic drainage and circulation- Moisturizes and improves skin elasticity, reducing the appearance of cellulite- Offers a relaxing, therapeutic experience that also benefits overall well-being

By incorporating castor oil body wraps into your wellness routine, you can enjoy the toning and detoxifying benefits of this natural remedy. This simple yet effective treatment not only aims to improve the appearance of your skin but also offers a moment of relaxation and self-care.

Overall Wellness and Longevity

Maximizing the potential of castor oil for overall wellness and longevity involves a holistic approach that extends beyond topical applications. This natural remedy, revered for centuries, offers a plethora of benefits that can enhance your health from the inside out. Here's how to incorporate castor oil into your wellness routine to support detoxification, hormonal balance, and vitality.

Detoxification and Lymphatic Drainage

Castor oil packs are a traditional and effective method for detoxifying the body and stimulating the lymphatic system. The lymphatic system, a crucial part of your immune system, helps remove toxins from your body. A sluggish lymphatic system can lead to a build-up of toxins, contributing to a host of health issues.- Materials Needed:- Cold-pressed castor oil- Wool flannel or cotton cloth- Plastic wrap- Hot water bottle or heating pad- Old towel- Instructions:

1. Soak the wool flannel or cotton cloth in castor oil until it is saturated but not dripping.

2. Place the soaked cloth over your abdomen, covering areas like the liver and intestines for a targeted detox effect.

3. Cover the cloth with plastic wrap to prevent staining and apply a hot water bottle or heating pad on top to facilitate the absorption of castor oil through the skin.

4. Relax with the pack in place for 30-60 minutes, allowing the castor oil to work its magic. This is an excellent opportunity for meditation or deep breathing exercises to further support relaxation and detoxification.

5. Repeat this process 1-3 times a week, depending on your detoxification goals and how your body responds.

Supporting Hormonal Balance

Hormonal imbalances can affect a wide range of bodily functions and contribute to various health issues. Castor oil packs, when applied to the lower abdomen, can support the health of the reproductive organs and help balance hormone levels, providing relief from menstrual discomfort and supporting reproductive health.- Instructions:

Follow the same steps as above, focusing the application on the lower abdomen. Consistent use, especially in the days leading up to menstruation, can help alleviate cramps and promote regular cycles.

Enhancing Energy and Vitality

Incorporating castor oil into your wellness routine can also boost energy levels and overall vitality. Its ability to support detoxification and hormonal balance indirectly contributes to enhanced energy by improving bodily functions and reducing the burden of toxins and hormonal disruptions.- Oral Consumption: While topical application is the most common method of using castor oil for health benefits, some practitioners recommend the cautious oral consumption of castor oil as a laxative to relieve constipation, which can also aid in detoxification. However, this should only be done under the guidance of a healthcare professional, as incorrect usage can lead to adverse effects.- Castor Oil in Diet: For a less direct approach, incorporating foods into your diet that naturally contain ricinoleic acid, the active component in castor oil, can also support health. While the castor bean itself is not safe to consume, focusing on a diet rich in anti-inflammatory and lymph-supportive foods can complement the external use of castor oil.

Safety Tips:- Always perform a patch test before using castor oil topically to ensure you do not have an allergic reaction.- Consult with a healthcare provider before using castor oil, especially if pregnant, nursing, or dealing with health conditions.

By integrating castor oil into your wellness practices, you can leverage its ancient healing properties to support your body's natural detoxification processes, balance hormones, and enhance your overall vitality. This natural remedy, used mindfully and consistently, can be a powerful tool in your journey towards holistic health and longevity.

Detoxification and Lymphatic Drainage

Harnessing the power of castor oil for detoxification and lymphatic drainage can be a transformative practice for enhancing your body's natural cleansing processes. This method leverages the unique properties of castor oil to support the lymphatic system, which plays a crucial role in removing toxins and waste from the body. Here's a step-by-step guide to performing a castor oil pack, a traditional and effective way to stimulate lymphatic drainage and detoxification.

Materials Needed:- Cold-pressed castor oil- Wool flannel or cotton cloth- Plastic wrap- Hot water bottle or heating pad- Old towel or sheet

Step-by-Step Instructions:

1. Prepare Your Space: Choose a comfortable area where you can lie down and relax for at least 30 to 60 minutes. Cover the area with an old towel or sheet to protect it from oil stains.

2. Soak the Cloth: Take the wool flannel or cotton cloth and soak it in cold-pressed castor oil. The cloth should be saturated but not dripping.

3. Apply the Cloth: Place the soaked cloth directly onto your skin, focusing on areas like the abdomen, which houses vital detoxification organs such as the liver and intestines.

4. Cover with Plastic Wrap: Use plastic wrap to cover the cloth. This helps to hold the cloth in place and prevents the oil from staining your clothing or furniture.

5. Apply Heat: Place a hot water bottle or heating pad over the plastic wrap. The heat generally help to increase the oil's penetration and stimulates the lymphatic system and the liver.

6. Relax: Lie down and relax with the pack in place for 30 to 60 minutes. This is an excellent opportu-

nity to practice deep breathing, meditation, or simply enjoy a quiet moment of relaxation.

7. Clean Up: After you have removed the pack, you can just cleanse the specific area with a diluted solution of water and baking soda. The cloth can be stored in a plastic bag in the refrigerator and reused for future applications.

Frequency of Use:

For optimal results, it's recommended to perform this procedure 1-3 times a week. Consistency is key to experiencing the full detoxifying benefits of castor oil packs.

Benefits:- Stimulates Lymphatic Drainage: Castor oil packs can help stimulate the flow of lymph, which carries waste products away from the tissues and supports the body's detoxification processes.- Supports Liver Function: The liver is your body's primary detoxification organ. Applying castor oil packs over the liver area can support liver function and enhance your body's ability to cleanse itself of toxins.- Reduces Inflammation: Castor oil has anti-inflammatory properties that can help reduce swelling and inflammation, further supporting detoxification and overall wellness.

Incorporating castor oil packs into your wellness routine can be a powerful way to support your body's natural detoxification processes, improve lymphatic health, and contribute to a sense of overall well-being.

Castor Oil for Hormonal Balance and Menopause Relief

Castor oil, with its unique composition, offers a natural pathway to support hormonal balance and provide relief during menopause. Its application through castor oil packs can be particularly beneficial in managing symptoms associated with hormonal fluctuations, such as hot flashes, mood swings, and sleep disturbances. Here's how to use castor oil packs for hormonal balance and menopause relief:

Materials Needed:- Cold-pressed castor oil- Wool flannel or cotton cloth- Plastic wrap- Hot water bottle or heating pad- Old towel

Instructions:

1. Soak the Cloth: Saturate the wool flannel or cotton cloth in cold-pressed castor oil. Ensure it is fully soaked but not excessively dripping.

2. Apply to Lower Abdomen: Place the soaked cloth over your lower abdomen. This area is targeted to support the reproductive organs and glands involved in hormonal regulation.

3. Secure with Plastic Wrap: Cover the cloth with plastic wrap. This helps to keep the pack in place and

enhances the absorption of castor oil into the skin.

4. Add Heat: Place a hot water bottle or heating pad over the plastic wrap. The heat aids in the penetration of castor oil and supports circulation to the area, which is essential for hormonal balance.

5. Relax: Lie down and relax with the pack in place for 30-60 minutes. This is an excellent opportunity to unwind, meditate, or read. The relaxation itself can further aid in balancing hormones, as stress reduction is key during menopause.

6. Repeat: For optimal results, use the castor oil pack 3-4 times a week. Consistency is crucial for seeing improvements in menopausal symptoms and hormonal balance.

Benefits:- Supports Detoxification: Castor oil packs help detoxify the liver, an organ that plays a vital role in regulating hormones, including estrogen levels.- Reduces Inflammation: The anti-inflammatory properties of castor oil can alleviate discomfort associated with menopause, such as joint pain and headaches.- Improves Lymphatic Circulation: Enhanced lymphatic drainage can support the removal of excess hormones and toxins from the body, contributing to hormonal balance.- Promotes Relaxation: The process of applying a castor oil pack encourages relaxation and stress relief, which is beneficial for managing mood swings and sleep issues during menopause.

Additional Tips:- Hydration: Drink plenty of water throughout the day to support the detoxification process initiated by castor oil packs.- Nutrition: Incorporate foods rich in phytoestrogens, such as flaxseeds and soy, which can help balance hormones naturally.- Exercise: Regular physical activity can help improving you mood, reduce the stress, and support the overall hormonal balance.

By integrating castor oil packs into your routine, you can harness a natural and effective method to support hormonal balance and alleviate menopausal symptoms, fostering a smoother transition through this natural phase of life.

Enhancing Energy and Vitality with Castor Oil

Castor oil, a natural remedy long cherished for its healing properties, also offers a unique benefit in boosting energy and vitality. Its ability to support lymphatic drainage, improve digestion, and balance hormones plays a crucial role in enhancing overall well-being and energy levels. Here's how to incorporate castor oil into your routine to tap into its vitality-enhancing benefits.

Materials Needed:- Cold-pressed castor oil- Wool flannel or cotton cloth- Plastic wrap- Hot water bottle or heating pad

Instructions for a Castor Oil Pack:

1. Soak the Cloth: Saturate the wool flannel or cotton cloth in cold-pressed castor oil. Ensure it's fully soaked but not dripping excessively.

2. Apply to the Abdomen: Place the soaked cloth over your abdomen. This area is targeted to support the digestive system and liver, key components in energy metabolism and detoxification.

3. Secure with Plastic Wrap: Cover the cloth with plastic wrap to keep it in place and maximize the absorption of castor oil through the skin.

4. Add Heat: Place a hot water bottle or heating pad over the plastic wrap. The added heat enhances the oil's penetration and stimulates blood circulation, aiding in the removal of toxins and supporting healthy digestion.

5. Relax: Lie down and relax with the pack in place for 30-60 minutes. This is an excellent opportunity to unwind and allow the castor oil pack to work effectively.

6. Frequency: For an energy boost, use the castor oil pack 2-3 times a week. Consistent use can help maintain optimal energy levels and support overall vitality.

Benefits:- Improved Digestion: By supporting the health of the digestive system, castor oil packs can aid in nutrient absorption and energy production, leading to increased vitality.- Detoxification: Regular use of castor oil packs helps in detoxifying the liver, a vital organ for energy metabolism and hormone balance. A well-functioning liver can significantly impact your energy levels and sense of well-being.- Hormonal Balance: Castor oil packs applied to the abdominal area can also support the glands responsible for hormone production, contributing to balanced energy levels throughout the day.- Stress Reduction: The process of applying a castor oil pack is inherently relaxing, helping to reduce stress levels. Lower stress levels contribute to improved energy and vitality, as the body conserves resources that would otherwise be expended in response to stress.

Additional Tips:- Stay Hydrated: Drinking plenty of water enhances the detoxifying effect of castor oil packs, further supporting energy levels.- Healthy Diet: A diet rich in whole foods, lean proteins, and healthy fats provides the necessary nutrients for sustained energy and vitality.- Regular Exercise: Incorporating regular physical activity into your routine can synergize with the benefits of castor oil, further enhancing energy levels and overall health.
By integrating castor oil packs into your wellness routine, you can harness its powerful benefits to boost your energy and vitality naturally. This simple yet effective practice supports key bodily functions that contribute to feeling energized and vibrant, offering a holistic approach to maintaining optimal health and well-being.

Book 6: Castor Oil for Digestive Health and Detox

Castor Oil Packs for Digestive Relief

Castor oil packs have been a cornerstone of natural health practices for centuries, particularly for their benefits in supporting digestive health and facilitating detoxification. The unique composition of castor oil, rich in ricinoleic acid, offers anti-inflammatory and lymphatic stimulating properties, making it an ideal remedy for a variety of digestive issues. Here's how to create and use castor oil packs for digestive relief:

Materials Needed:- Cold-pressed castor oil- Wool flannel or cotton cloth- Plastic wrap- Hot water bottle or heating pad- Old towel

Step-by-Step Instructions:

1. Soak the Cloth: Begin by soaking the wool flannel or cotton cloth in cold-pressed castor oil. Ensure the cloth is saturated but not excessively dripping to avoid mess.

2. Apply to Abdomen: Place the soaked cloth over your abdomen, targeting areas where you experience discomfort. This could be the lower abdomen for issues like IBS or constipation, or the upper abdomen for concerns related to the liver and gallbladder.

3. Cover with Plastic Wrap: Use plastic wrap to cover the cloth, securing it in place and preventing oil from staining your clothing or furniture.

4. Add Heat: Position a hot water bottle or heating pad over the plastic wrap. The heat aids in the absorption of the oil and further stimulates the lymphatic and digestive systems.

5. Rest and Relax: Lie down and relax with the pack in place for 45-60 minutes. This is an excellent opportunity to meditate, listen to soothing music, or simply rest.

6. Clean Up: After removing the pack, you can try to clean the area with a diluted solution of water and baking soda to remove the residual oil. The cloth can be stored in a plastic bag in the refrigerator and reused for future applications.

Frequency of Use:

For digestive issues, using the castor oil pack 2-3 times a week can provide significant relief. Consistency is key, as the benefits accumulate over time.

Benefits:- Supports Digestive Function: Castor oil packs can help stimulate digestion, relieve constipation, and reduce bloating by enhancing the function of the digestive organs.- Detoxification: The packs support liver function, a key organ in the body's detoxification process, helping to cleanse the body of toxins that can contribute to digestive discomfort.- Reduces Inflammation: The anti-inflammatory properties of castor oil can soothe inflamed digestive tracts, providing relief from conditions like IBS and Crohn's disease.

Gut Healing and Inflammation Reduction

Inflammation in the gut can lead to a host of issues, from acute discomfort to chronic health conditions. Castor oil's anti-inflammatory properties make it a valuable tool in healing the gut and reducing inflammation. Incorporating castor oil internally should be done with caution and under the guidance of a healthcare professional, as its laxative effect can be strong. However, topical application through packs, as described, is safe and beneficial for most individuals.

Supporting Healthy Digestion:- Diet: Complement castor oil packs with a diet rich in fiber, probiotics, and anti-inflammatory foods to enhance digestive health.- Hydration: Adequate water intake is crucial for maintaining healthy digestion and facilitating the body's natural detoxification processes.- Stress Management: Stress can significantly impact digestive health. Practices such as yoga, meditation, and deep breathing can help manage stress and improve overall digestive function.

By integrating castor oil packs into your routine, you can support your digestive health naturally, reducing discomfort and enhancing your body's detoxification processes. This simple, yet effective remedy offers a holistic approach to managing digestive issues and promoting overall well-being.

Castor Oil Packs for Digestive Relief

Creating and using castor oil packs for digestive relief is a gentle, yet powerful way to address a variety of digestive issues, from bloating and constipation to more chronic conditions like irritable bowel syndrome (IBS) and inflammation. The process harnesses the anti-inflammatory and lymphatic-stimulating properties of castor oil, providing a soothing, natural remedy that promotes healing and supports overall digestive health.

Materials Needed:- Cold-pressed castor oil- Wool flannel or cotton cloth- Plastic wrap- Hot water bottle or heating pad- Old towel or sheet

Step-by-Step Instructions:

1. Prepare the Area: Choose a comfortable, quiet space where you can lie down and relax. Protect the surface with an old towel or sheet to catch any potential oil drips.

2. Soak the Cloth: Take your wool flannel or cotton cloth and saturate it with cold-pressed castor oil. The cloth should be wet but not dripping excessively.

3. Apply the Cloth: Place the oil-soaked cloth directly onto your abdomen, covering the area that corresponds with your digestive discomfort. For general digestive health, covering the entire abdomen is recommended.

4. Wrap with Plastic: Cover the cloth with plastic wrap. This helps to keep the castor oil in place and increases its effectiveness by ensuring it doesn't evaporate or rub off on clothing or furniture.

5. Apply Heat: Place a hot water bottle or heating pad over the plastic wrap. The heat will aid in the absorption of the castor oil into the skin and help to relax the muscles of the digestive tract, enhancing the oil's therapeutic effects.

6. Rest: Lie down and relax with the pack in place for at least 45-60 minutes. This is an excellent opportunity to practice deep breathing, meditate, or simply rest. The relaxation will further aid digestion and the healing process.

7. Clean Up: After removing the pack, you can clean your skin with a simple solution of water and baking soda to remove any residual oil. The cloth can be stored in a plastic bag in the refrigerator and reused for future applications.

Frequency of Use:

For chronic conditions or severe discomfort, using the castor oil pack 3-4 times a week can provide significant relief and promote healing. For maintenance of digestive health or mild issues, 1-2 times a week may be sufficient.

Benefits:- Enhanced Digestive Function: Castor oil packs can help stimulate digestion, relieve constipation, and reduce bloating by enhancing the function of the digestive organs.- Detoxification Support: The packs support liver function, aiding the body's natural detoxification processes and helping to cleanse the digestive tract of toxins and waste.- Inflammation Reduction: The anti-inflammatory properties of castor oil can soothe an inflamed digestive tract, providing relief from conditions like IBS, Crohn's disease, and colitis.- Stress Reduction: The process of applying a castor oil pack is inherently relaxing, helping to reduce stress levels, which are often a contributing factor to digestive issues.

Incorporating castor oil packs into your wellness routine can be a simple yet effective way to support digestive health, relieve discomfort, and promote a balanced, functioning digestive system.

How to Make and Use Castor Oil Packs

To harness the therapeutic benefits of castor oil for digestive relief and detoxification, creating and using castor oil packs is a time-honored method. This process involves applying a cloth soaked in castor oil to the abdomen, which can help enhance circulation, promote healing, and support the body's natural detox processes. Here's a detailed guide to making and using castor oil packs effectively.

Materials Needed:- High-quality, cold-pressed castor oil- A piece of wool flannel or cotton cloth large enough to cover the abdominal area- Plastic wrap or a large plastic bag- A heating pad or hot water bottle- An old towel or sheet to protect bedding or furniture- Safety pins or clips (optional, for securing the cloth)

Step-by-Step Instructions:

1. Prepare the Area: Choose a comfortable, quiet place where you can lie down and relax. Spread an old towel or sheet to protect the surface from oil stains.

2. Soak the Cloth: Take the wool flannel or cotton cloth and fold it into two or three layers to fit over your entire abdomen. Soak the cloth in castor oil until it is completely saturated but is not dripping. You may warm the oil slightly to enhance the soothing effect, but ensure it is not too hot to avoid burns.

3. Apply the Cloth to Your Abdomen: Place the soaked cloth directly on your skin, covering the abdominal area. The liver is located on the right side of the body, so ensure this area is well covered if you're focusing on liver detoxification.

4. Cover with Plastic: Wrap the plastic wrap or place the plastic bag over the cloth to prevent the oil from seeping into your clothing or furniture. The plastic also helps to hold in warmth, which aids in the absorption of the castor oil.

5. Apply Heat: Place a small heating pad or a hot water bottle over the plastic wrap. The heat will help the castor oil penetrate more deeply into the skin and underlying tissues, enhancing its therapeutic effects. Keep the heat source in place for at least 45-60 minutes. If using a heating pad, ensure it's set to a comfortable temperature to avoid overheating.

6. Relax: Lie back and relax while the castor oil pack does its work. You might listen to soothing music, meditate, or simply rest. This is an excellent time for introspection or relaxation, as the pack's benefits are enhanced by a calm, stress-free state.

7. Remove and Cleanse: After the recommended time, remove the pack and cleanse the area with a warm, damp cloth. You can also mix a little baking soda with water for a gentle cleansing solution that helps remove any residual oil.

8. Store for Reuse: The same castor oil-soaked cloth can be reused multiple times. Fold the cloth, place it in a plastic bag, and store it in the refrigerator. Before each use, add more castor oil as needed to

keep it well saturated.

Frequency of Use:

For general wellness and detoxification, using a castor oil pack 2-3 times a week is recommended. For specific issues or under the guidance of a healthcare professional, the frequency may vary.

Benefits:- Supports lymphatic circulation, aiding in the removal of toxins- Promotes relaxation and reduces inflammation- Enhances liver function and digestive health

By incorporating castor oil packs into your wellness routine, you can take advantage of the oil's natural healing properties to support your body's detoxification processes and improve overall digestive health.

Healing Benefits for IBS, Constipation, and Bloating

For individuals grappling with IBS, constipation, and bloating, castor oil emerges as a gentle yet potent natural remedy. Its unique composition, particularly the presence of ricinoleic acid, offers anti-inflammatory and laxative properties that can soothe the digestive tract and promote regular bowel movements. Here's how to leverage castor oil for digestive relief:

Castor Oil Application for Constipation Relief:- Materials Needed:- Pure, cold-pressed castor oil- Cotton pad or clean cloth- Instructions:

1. Warm a tablespoon of castor oil by placing the oil container in a bowl of hot water for a few minutes. Ensure the oil is comfortably warm to the touch, not hot.

2. Soak a cotton pad or clean cloth in the warm castor oil.

3. Apply the soaked pad directly to the abdomen, focusing on the lower belly area where the colon is located.

4. Gently massage the area in a clockwise direction. This motion aligns with the natural movement of the colon, aiding in the stimulation of bowel movements.

5. For enhanced absorption, cover the area with a warm cloth or heating pad for 20-30 minutes.

6. Practice this routine nightly before bed to help regulate bowel movements.

Castor Oil Packs for IBS and Bloating:- Materials Needed:- Cold-pressed castor oil- Wool flannel or cotton cloth- Plastic wrap- Hot water bottle or heating pad- Old towel- Instructions:

1. Saturate the wool flannel or cotton cloth in castor oil until it is fully soaked but not dripping.

2. Place the soaked cloth on the abdomen, covering the entire area affected by IBS symptoms or bloating.

3. Cover the cloth with plastic wrap to prevent oil from leaking onto clothing or bedding.

4. Place a hot water bottle or heating pad over the plastic wrap to help the castor oil penetrate deeper into the skin.

5. Lie down and relax with the pack in place for 45-60 minutes. This is an ideal time to rest or meditate, allowing the body to heal.

6. Repeat this process 2-3 times a week, especially during flare-ups of IBS or episodes of severe bloating, to reduce symptoms.

Dietary Considerations:

While castor oil provides external support, addressing dietary triggers is crucial for long-term relief from IBS, constipation, and bloating. Incorporating fiber-rich foods, staying hydrated, and avoiding known irritants like dairy, gluten, or high-FODMAP foods can complement the healing effects of castor oil.

Safety Tips:- Always conduct a patch test before applying castor oil to the skin to ensure no allergic reactions occur.- Consult with a healthcare provider before starting any new treatment, especially if you have a medical condition or are pregnant.

By integrating castor oil into your wellness routine, you can harness its natural healing properties to provide relief from the discomforts of IBS, constipation, and bloating. This, combined with mindful dietary habits, can significantly improve digestive health and overall well-being.

Liver Cleansing and Detoxification

The liver, a vital organ for detoxification and metabolism, benefits significantly from the application of castor oil packs. This method enhances the liver's ability to cleanse the blood, break down toxins, and support overall digestive health. Here's a guide to using castor oil packs for liver cleansing and detoxification:

Materials Needed:- Cold-pressed castor oil- Wool flannel or cotton cloth- Plastic wrap- Hot water bottle or heating pad- Old towel

Instructions:

1. Soak the Cloth: Fully saturate the wool flannel or cotton cloth with cold-pressed castor oil. The cloth should be wet but not dripping, to ensure a mess-free application.

2. Position the Cloth: Place the oil-soaked cloth over the right side of your abdomen, where the liver is located, just below the rib cage. This direct application targets the liver area, facilitating detoxification.

3. Secure with Plastic Wrap: Cover the cloth with plastic wrap. This step is crucial as it prevents the oil from staining your clothes or furniture and helps maintain the cloth's position over the liver area.

4. Apply Heat: Place a hot water bottle or heating pad over the plastic wrap. The heat aids in the deeper penetration of castor oil into the skin and stimulates the liver and gallbladder, promoting detoxification and increasing lymphatic circulation.

5. Relax and Detoxify: Lie down and relax with the pack in place for 45-60 minutes. This duration allows ample time for the castor oil to work on stimulating liver function and supporting the body's natural detox pathways.

6. Remove and Clean: After the time is up, remove the pack and cleanse the area with a warm, damp cloth. You can also use a mixture of water and baking soda for a gentle cleanse that removes any residual oil.

7. Reuse and Store: The same castor oil-soaked cloth can be reused several times. Store it in a plastic bag in the refrigerator between uses. Before each use, add more castor oil to keep it well saturated.

Frequency of Use:

For effective liver detoxification, using the castor oil pack 2-3 times a week is recommended. Consistent use over time supports liver health and enhances the body's natural detoxification processes.

Benefits:- Enhanced Liver Function: The application of castor oil packs over the liver area helps in improving liver function, crucial for detoxifying the body.- Stimulation of Lymphatic Drainage: Castor oil packs promote lymphatic circulation, which is essential for removing toxins from the body and supporting immune function.- Reduction of Inflammation: The anti-inflammatory properties of castor oil can help reduce inflammation in the liver and surrounding tissues, supporting healing and function.- Support for Digestive Health: By improving liver function, castor oil packs indirectly support digestive health, contributing to better nutrient absorption and metabolism.

Integrating castor oil packs into your routine for liver cleansing and detoxification can offer a simple yet effective natural remedy to support liver health and enhance your body's detoxification capabilities.

Gut Healing and Inflammation Reduction

Gut health is foundational to overall wellness, influencing everything from digestion and absorption of nutrients to immune function and even mood regulation. Inflammation in the gut can disrupt this delicate balance, leading to a myriad of health issues. Fortunately, natural remedies like castor oil offer a gentle yet effective approach to healing the gut and reducing inflammation. Here's how to incorporate castor oil into your gut health regimen:

Castor Oil Packs for Gut Health

Castor oil packs, applied externally, can significantly impact gut health by enhancing circulation, promoting lymphatic drainage, and reducing inflammation. This method is particularly beneficial for conditions such as leaky gut syndrome, IBS, and general digestive discomfort.- Materials Needed:- Cold-pressed castor oil- Wool flannel or cotton cloth- Plastic wrap- Hot water bottle or heating pad- Old towel- Instructions:

1. Soak the wool flannel or cotton cloth in castor oil until it is saturated but not dripping.

2. Place the cloth over your abdomen, covering the entire gut area.

3. Cover with plastic wrap to prevent oil from leaking onto clothing or bedding.

4. Place a hot water bottle or heating pad over the plastic wrap to help the castor oil penetrate more deeply.

5. Relax with the pack in place for 45-60 minutes, allowing the anti-inflammatory properties of the oil to work.

6. Repeat 2-3 times a week for best results.

Dietary Adjustments to Support Gut Healing

In addition to external applications of castor oil, addressing dietary factors is crucial for gut healing. Incorporating anti-inflammatory foods and avoiding gut irritants can complement the healing effects of castor oil packs.- Incorporate Anti-inflammatory Foods:- Omega-3 rich foods like salmon, chia seeds, and walnuts- Fermented foods for probiotics, such as yogurt, kefir, and sauerkraut- High-fiber foods, including vegetables, fruits, and whole grains, to support healthy digestion- Avoid Gut Irritants:- Processed and sugary foods that can exacerbate inflammation- Common allergens like gluten and dairy, if sensitive- Excessive alcohol and caffeine, which can disrupt gut flora and irritate the gut lining

Lifestyle Modifications for Enhanced Gut Health

The healing process is holistic, involving more than just diet and remedies. Incorporating lifestyle changes can further support gut health and reduce inflammation.- Manage Stress:

Chronic stress can negatively affect gut health. Practices such as yoga or meditation can also help you manage stress levels.- Ensure Adequate Sleep:

Quality sleep is crucial for healing and inflammation reduction. Aim for 7-9 hours of restful sleep per night.- Stay Hydrated:

Adequate hydration supports digestion and helps flush toxins from the body. Aim for at least 8 glasses of water daily.- Exercise Regularly:

Regular physical activity can improve digestion, reduce stress, and support overall gut health.

By combining the external application of castor oil packs with dietary adjustments and lifestyle modifications, you can create a comprehensive approach to healing the gut and reducing inflammation. This holistic strategy not only addresses the symptoms but also targets the underlying causes of gut health issues, promoting long-term wellness and vitality.

Castor Oil and Gut-Brain Health Connection

The connection between the gut and the brain, often referred to as the gut-brain axis, is a complex communication network that links the emotional and cognitive centers of the brain with peripheral intestinal functions. Emerging research highlights the pivotal role of this connection in overall health and well-being, with castor oil playing a supportive role in enhancing gut health and, by extension, influencing brain health.

Castor oil, known for its potent anti-inflammatory and antibacterial properties, can be a valuable tool in managing gut health, which in turn impacts the gut-brain axis. The primary component of castor oil, ricinoleic acid, has been shown to promote smooth muscle contraction in the intestines, helping to facilitate bowel movements and detoxification. This action can alleviate constipation, a common issue that can affect mood and cognitive function due to the discomfort and toxicity it causes.

Moreover, the anti-inflammatory properties of castor oil can help soothe irritated digestive tracts, reducing gut inflammation which is often linked to mood disorders such as anxiety and depression. Inflammation in the gut can send signals to the brain that trigger mood changes, highlighting the importance of maintaining gut health for mental well-being.

To harness the benefits of castor oil for the gut-brain health connection, consider the following application method:

1. Topical Application: Apply a castor oil pack to the abdomen to support digestion and promote a healthy inflammatory response. Soak a piece of wool flannel in castor oil, place it on the abdomen, cover with plastic wrap, and apply a heat source such as a hot water bottle for 45-60 minutes. This method can help stimulate the lymphatic system, reduce inflammation, and promote healing in the gut, thereby supporting the gut-brain axis.

2. Dietary Considerations: While the direct ingestion of castor oil for gut health should only be considered under the guidance of a healthcare professional due to its potent laxative effects, incorporating anti-inflammatory foods and probiotics into your diet can complement the benefits of topical castor oil applications. Foods rich in omega-3 fatty acids, fiber, and fermented foods can support gut health and, consequently, brain health.

3. Hydration: Adequate hydration is crucial for maintaining the mucosal lining of the intestines, facilitating the removal of toxins, and supporting overall digestive health. Drinking sufficient water daily can enhance the effectiveness of castor oil treatments by aiding in detoxification and ensuring smooth bowel movements.

4. Stress Management: Techniques such as meditation, yoga, and deep breathing exercises can help manage stress, which is known to have a profound impact on gut health. Reducing stress through these practices can enhance the gut-brain connection, improving both digestive and mental health.

By integrating castor oil into a holistic approach that includes dietary adjustments, adequate hydration, and stress management techniques, individuals can support their gut-brain health connection. This comprehensive strategy not only aids in maintaining digestive comfort but also promotes mental clarity, mood stability, and overall well-being.

Anti-Inflammatory Gut Healing Elixirs

Crafting anti-inflammatory gut healing elixirs with castor oil can be a transformative addition to your wellness routine, offering a natural approach to soothing digestive discomfort and enhancing gut health. These elixirs leverage the anti-inflammatory properties of castor oil in combination with other gut-friendly ingredients to create powerful drinks that support healing and reduce inflammation. Here are two recipes to get you started:

1. Castor Oil and Turmeric Elixir

Ingredients:- 1 teaspoon of cold-pressed castor oil- 1 cup of warm almond milk or coconut milk- ½ teaspoon of turmeric powder- A pinch of black pepper (to enhance turmeric absorption)- 1 teaspoon of honey or maple syrup (optional, for sweetness)

Instructions:

1. Warm the almond or coconut milk in a saucepan over low heat until it is just warm to the touch. Avoid boiling to preserve the nutrients.

2. Transfer the warm milk to a mug and stir in the turmeric powder and black pepper.

3. Add the cold-pressed castor oil and sweetener of your choice. Stir well to combine all the ingredients.

4. Drink this elixir in the evening, a few hours before bedtime, to allow the anti-inflammatory properties to work overnight.

5. Castor Oil and Ginger Digestive Soothe

Ingredients:- 1 teaspoon of cold-pressed castor oil- 1 cup of hot water- ½ teaspoon of freshly grated ginger- Juice of half a lemon- 1 teaspoon of raw honey (optional, for sweetness)

Instructions:

1. Pour hot water into a mug and add the freshly grated ginger. Allow it to steep for 3-5 minutes.

2. Strain the ginger pieces from the water and return the ginger-infused water to the mug.

3. Stir in the lemon juice and cold-pressed castor oil. Mix well to ensure the oil is well integrated.

4. Add honey if desired and stir until dissolved.

5. Enjoy this elixir in the morning on an empty stomach to kickstart your digestive system and reduce inflammation throughout the day.

Benefits:- Turmeric is renowned for its potent anti-inflammatory and antioxidant properties, making it an ideal companion to castor oil for gut health.- Ginger has been used for centuries to soothe digestive issues, reduce nausea, and support immune health.- Lemon provides vitamin C and aids in digestion and detoxification.- Black Pepper increases the bioavailability of curcumin, the active compound in turmeric, enhancing its absorption and effectiveness.- Honey offers antimicrobial benefits and can soothe the digestive tract, in addition to providing a natural sweetness to the elixirs.

These elixirs are designed to be a part of a balanced approach to gut health, complementing a diet rich in whole foods, fiber, and probiotics. Regular consumption can help soothe the digestive system, reduce inflammation, and support overall wellness. Remember, while castor oil is beneficial for its anti-inflammatory properties, it's important to use it in moderation and consult with a healthcare provider if you have any underlying health conditions or concerns.

Treating Leaky Gut Syndrome and Ulcers

Leaky Gut Syndrome and ulcers, conditions that significantly impact digestive health, can be addressed through a holistic approach incorporating castor oil, known for its healing and anti-inflammatory properties. Here's a guide to using castor oil as part of a regimen to soothe and repair the gut lining, offering relief from these conditions.

Castor Oil Packs for Gut Healing

Castor oil packs, applied externally, can aid in the healing process of the gut by reducing inflammation and promoting tissue repair. The ricinoleic acid in castor oil serves as a potent anti-inflammatory agent, making it beneficial for those suffering from Leaky Gut Syndrome and ulcers.- Materials Needed:- Cold-pressed castor oil- Wool flannel or cotton cloth- Plastic wrap- Hot water bottle or heating pad- Old towel- Application Process:

1. Soak the wool flannel or cotton cloth in castor oil until it is saturated but not dripping.

2. Place the cloth directly on the abdomen, targeting the area where the gut inflammation or ulcers are most problematic.

3. Cover with plastic wrap to prevent oil from leaking onto clothing or bedding.

4. Place a hot water bottle or heating pad over the plastic wrap to enhance the oil's penetration through the skin.

5. Relax with the pack in place for 45-60 minutes to allow the anti-inflammatory properties of the oil to work.

6. Practice this routine 3-4 times a week to support healing of the gut lining and relief from discomfort.

Dietary Adjustments to Support Healing

In conjunction with castor oil packs, dietary adjustments play a crucial role in healing Leaky Gut Syndrome and ulcers. Incorporating anti-inflammatory foods and eliminating gut irritants can accelerate the healing process.- Foods to Include:- Bone broth, rich in collagen, which helps repair the gut lining.- Fermented foods like kefir, sauerkraut, and kimchi, which introduce beneficial probiotics.- Healthy fats, such as coconut oil and avocados, to reduce inflammation.- Foods to Avoid:- Processed foods and sugars that can exacerbate inflammation and irritation.- Gluten and dairy, if sensitivity is present, as they can trigger immune responses harming the gut.- Alcohol and caffeine, which can irritate the gut lining and disrupt the healing process.

Lifestyle Modifications for Enhanced Gut Health- Stress Management: Chronic stress can weaken the gut lining and slow the healing process. Techniques such as yoga, meditation, and deep breathing exercises can help manage stress effectively.- Adequate Sleep: Ensuring 7-9 hours of quality sleep per night supports the body's natural healing processes.- Hydration: Drinking sufficient water daily aids in detoxification and maintains mucosal lining health.

Monitoring and Adjustments- Listen to Your Body: Pay attention to how your body responds to different foods and adjust your diet accordingly.- Consult Healthcare Providers: Regular check-ins with healthcare professionals can help monitor the healing process and adjust treatments as necessary.

By integrating castor oil packs with dietary and lifestyle changes, individuals suffering from Leaky Gut Syndrome and ulcers can find relief and promote long-term gut health. This holistic approach addresses the root causes of these conditions, supporting the body's natural healing capabilities.

Weight Loss and Metabolism Boost

Supporting Healthy Weight Loss with Castor Oil

Castor oil, renowned for its anti-inflammatory and antimicrobial properties, also plays a supportive role in weight loss and metabolism enhancement. When combined with a balanced diet and regular exercise, castor oil can help improve digestive efficiency, detoxify the body, and stimulate lymphatic drainage, contributing to a healthier metabolism and aiding in weight management.

Castor Oil Packs for Metabolic Support- Materials Needed:- Cold-pressed castor oil- Wool flannel or cotton cloth- Plastic wrap- Hot water bottle or heating pad- Old towel- Application Process:

1. Saturate the wool flannel or cotton cloth with cold-pressed castor oil, ensuring it is fully soaked but not dripping.

2. Place the cloth over the abdomen to target the liver and digestive organs, areas crucial for metabolism and detoxification.

3. Cover the cloth with plastic wrap to prevent oil leakage and secure it in place.

4. Apply a hot water bottle or heating pad over the plastic wrap to enhance the absorption of castor oil into the skin.

5. Relax with the pack in place for 45-60 minutes, allowing the castor oil to stimulate the liver, aid in detoxification, and support metabolic functions.

6. Perform this routine 2-3 times a week to support metabolism and assist in weight loss efforts.

Recipes for Metabolism-Boosting Castor Oil Smoothies

Incorporating castor oil into your diet through smoothies can provide an internal boost to your metabolism. Here are two recipes designed to enhance metabolic rate and support weight loss:

1. Green Detox Smoothie- Ingredients:- 1 teaspoon of cold-pressed castor oil- 1 cup of spinach or kale- 1/2 green apple, chopped- 1/2 avocado- 1 tablespoon of chia seeds- 1 cup of almond milk or water- Ice cubes (optional)- Instructions:

1. Combine all ingredients in a small blender.

2. Blend until it gets smooth and creamy.

3. Enjoy this smoothie in the morning to kickstart your metabolism and provide energy throughout the day.

4. Berry Metabolism Booster

Ingredients:- 1 teaspoon of cold-pressed castor oil- 1 cup of mixed berries (strawberries, blueberries, raspberries)- 1 banana- 1 tablespoon of flaxseeds- 1 cup of Greek yogurt or kefir- Ice cubes (optional)- Instructions:

1. Place all ingredients in a blender.

2. Blend until smooth.

3. Drink this berry smoothie as a nutritious snack or breakfast to support metabolism and aid in weight management.

Castor Oil Wraps for Targeted Fat Reduction

While not a substitute for healthy diet and exercise, castor oil wraps can complement weight loss efforts by targeting specific areas for fat reduction, such as the thighs, abdomen, and arms.- Materials Needed:- Cold-pressed castor oil- Plastic wrap- Warm towel or heating pad- Application Process:

1. Apply a generous amount of cold-pressed castor oil to the targeted area.

2. Wrap the area with plastic wrap to secure the oil.

3. Apply a warm towel or heating pad for 30-45 minutes to enhance absorption.

4. Use this method 2-3 times a week to support localized fat reduction and skin tightening.

By integrating castor oil into your wellness routine through topical applications, dietary inclusions, and targeted wraps, you can support your weight loss journey and boost your metabolism. Remember, consistency and a holistic approach to health and wellness are key to achieving and maintaining your weight loss goals.

Supporting Healthy Weight Loss with Castor Oil

Castor oil, a natural remedy with a rich history of medicinal use, offers unique benefits that can support healthy weight loss efforts. Its ability to enhance digestion, improve lymphatic circulation, and boost metabolism makes it a valuable addition to a holistic weight management plan. Here's how to incorporate castor oil into your routine to aid in achieving a healthier weight:

1. Enhance Digestive Efficiency: Regular use of castor oil packs on the abdomen can stimulate the digestive system, promoting better nutrient absorption and reducing issues such as bloating and constipation. Improved digestion directly supports weight loss by ensuring that food is processed more efficiently, reducing the likelihood of fat storage.

   - Materials Needed: Cold-pressed castor oil, wool flannel or cotton cloth, plastic wrap, hot water bottle or heating pad.

   - Application: Soak the cloth in castor oil, place it over the abdomen, cover with plastic wrap, and apply heat for 45-60 minutes. This process can be done 2-3 times a week.

2. Stimulate Lymphatic Drainage: The lymphatic system plays a crucial role in detoxifying the body and maintaining immune function. Castor oil packs applied to different areas of the body can stimulate lymphatic flow, aiding in the removal of toxins and excess fluids that can contribute to weight gain.

3. Boost Metabolism: The topical application of castor oil may also have a thermogenic effect, slightly increasing the body's temperature and, consequently, its metabolic rate. This means the body burns more calories, even at rest, which can aid in weight loss.

4. Incorporate into a Balanced Diet: While castor oil should not be ingested as a weight loss supplement due to its strong laxative properties, focusing on a balanced diet rich in whole foods, lean proteins, and healthy fats, alongside regular castor oil pack use, can support metabolic health and

weight loss.

5. Combine with Regular Exercise: No weight loss strategy is complete without physical activity. Combining the use of castor oil packs with a consistent exercise routine can enhance fat burning, improve muscle tone, and contribute to overall weight loss.

6. Stay Hydrated: Drinking plenty of water is essential for weight loss and overall health. Water helps to flush toxins from the body, supports efficient metabolism, and can reduce hunger, often confused with thirst.

7. Get Adequate Sleep: Quality sleep is crucial for weight management. Lack of sleep can disrupt hormones that regulate appetite, leading to increased hunger and potential weight gain. Aim for 7-9 hours of restful sleep per night.

8. Manage Stress: High stress levels can lead to weight gain by affecting appetite and food choices. Incorporating stress-reduction techniques such as meditation, yoga, or deep breathing exercises can help manage stress and support weight loss efforts.

By integrating castor oil into a comprehensive approach that includes diet, exercise, hydration, sleep, and stress management, individuals can support healthy weight loss and improve overall well-being. Remember, consistency and a holistic lifestyle are key to achieving and maintaining weight loss goals.

Recipes for Metabolism-Boosting Castor Oil Smoothies

Boosting your metabolism can significantly enhance your weight loss efforts and overall energy levels. Incorporating castor oil into your diet through smoothies is a creative and effective way to enjoy its health benefits. Here are two delicious smoothie recipes designed to kickstart your metabolism and support your wellness journey.

1. Castor Oil Citrus Blast

Ingredients:- 1 teaspoon of cold-pressed castor oil- 1 cup of fresh orange juice- ½ grapefruit, juiced- ½ lemon, juiced- ½ inch of fresh ginger, peeled and minced- A pinch of cayenne pepper- Ice cubes (optional)

Instructions:

1. Combine the orange juice, grapefruit juice, lemon juice, and minced ginger in a blender.

2. Add the teaspoon of cold-pressed castor oil and a pinch of cayenne pepper to the mixture. The cayenne pepper not only adds a kick but also works to boost your metabolism further.

3. Blend until smooth. If you prefer a colder drink, feel free to add ice cubes and blend until you reach your desired consistency.

4. Enjoy this citrus blast first thing in the morning to awaken your digestive system and jumpstart your metabolism for the day.

5. Green Metabolism Booster

Ingredients:- 1 teaspoon of cold-pressed castor oil- 1 cup of unsweetened almond milk- 1 cup of spinach leaves- ½ cucumber, chopped- ½ avocado- 1 tablespoon of chia seeds- 1 apple, cored and sliced- Ice cubes (optional)

Instructions:

1. Place the spinach leaves, chopped cucumber, avocado, and apple slices into the blender.

2. Add the unsweetened almond milk and a teaspoon of cold-pressed castor oil to the mix. The avocado adds creaminess and healthy fats, which are essential for absorbing the nutrients in the smoothie.

3. Sprinkle the tablespoon of chia seeds into the blender. Chia seeds are not only a great source of fiber but also help to keep you feeling full longer.

4. Blend all the ingredients until smooth. For a chilled version, add ice cubes to your preference.

5. Drink this smoothie as a meal replacement or a mid-day snack to fuel your body and boost your metabolism.

These smoothie recipes incorporate castor oil in a way that complements the natural flavors of the other ingredients while providing a metabolism-boosting effect. Regular consumption of these smoothies, alongside a balanced diet and exercise routine, can help support your body's natural processes and contribute to your overall health and wellness goals. Remember, when using castor oil, always opt for cold-pressed, hexane-free oil to ensure you're getting the highest quality product.

Castor Oil Wraps for Targeted Fat Reduction

Castor Oil Wraps for Targeted Fat Reduction offer a unique method to complement your weight loss journey. By focusing on specific areas, these wraps can help in the reduction of fat accumulation, improve skin elasticity, and enhance circulation. Here's how to effectively use castor oil wraps for targeting areas like the abdomen, thighs, and arms.

Materials Needed:- High-quality, cold-pressed castor oil- Plastic wrap- Wool flannel or cotton cloth-
Warm towel or heating pad- Bandage wrap or a tight-fitting garment

Step-by-Step Instructions:

1. Prepare the Skin: Start with clean, slightly damp skin. This helps in the better absorption of castor oil.

2. Apply Castor Oil: Generously apply cold-pressed castor oil to the target area. Ensure that the area is fully covered with a thin layer of oil.

3. Place the Cloth: Put the wool flannel or cotton cloth over the oiled skin. This cloth acts as a medium to hold the oil against your skin and prevent direct contact with the plastic wrap.

4. Wrap with Plastic: Carefully wrap the plastic wrap around the cloth-covered area. The plastic wrap should be snug but not too tight to avoid discomfort.

5. Apply Heat: Place a warm towel or heating pad over the wrapped area. The heat helps in opening the pores and allows for deeper penetration of castor oil into the skin.

6. Secure the Wrap: If needed, use a bandage wrap or wear a tight-fitting garment over the plastic wrap to keep everything in place. This is particularly useful if you plan to move around.

7. Relaxation Time: Sit back and relax for at least 45-60 minutes. This is a great time to read, meditate, or simply unwind as the castor oil wrap does its work.

8. Removal and Clean Up: Carefully remove the plastic wrap and cloth. Wipe off any excess oil with a warm, damp towel. If desired, follow up with a gentle massage to enhance circulation.

9. Frequency: For best results, use the castor oil wraps 2-3 times a week. Consistency is key to seeing targeted fat reduction and skin improvement.

Benefits:- Detoxification: Castor oil is known for its ability to draw out toxins, which can contribute to fat accumulation.- Improved Circulation: The process helps in boosting blood flow to the targeted area, aiding in the breakdown of fat cells.- Skin Tightening: Regular use can lead to firmer, more elastic skin, reducing the appearance of cellulite.

Safety Tips:- Always perform a patch test to ensure you do not have an allergic reaction to castor oil.- Do not apply castor oil wraps on broken or irritated skin.- Pregnant women should consult with a healthcare provider before using castor oil wraps.

Incorporating Castor Oil Wraps into your wellness routine can be an effective way to target stubborn fat areas, improve skin texture, and support overall body detoxification. Remember, while castor oil wraps can aid in fat reduction, they should be used in conjunction with a balanced diet and regular exercise for optimal results.

Conclusion - Empowering Your Natural Beauty Journey with Castor Oil Key Takeaways and Next Steps:

Empowering your journey towards natural beauty and wellness with castor oil marks a significant step in embracing holistic health practices. The versatility and efficacy of castor oil, as explored throughout this guide, offer a foundation for incorporating this ancient remedy into various aspects of your daily life. From enhancing the radiance of your skin and the luster of your hair to supporting digestive health and providing natural solutions for family wellness, castor oil stands as a testament to the power of natural remedies.

Building Your Castor Oil Beauty and Wellness Routine involves understanding the unique needs of your skin and hair, as well as recognizing the broader applications of castor oil in your wellness practices. Start by integrating castor oil into your skincare and haircare routines gradually, paying attention to how your body responds. Experiment with the DIY recipes provided, adjusting ingredients as needed to suit your personal preferences and specific concerns. Remember, consistency is key to seeing tangible benefits, so incorporate castor oil treatments into your regular self-care rituals.

Continuing Your Journey Towards Radiant Health and Timeless Beauty means staying curious and open to learning. The world of natural health and beauty is ever-evolving, with ongoing research shedding light on new uses and benefits of traditional remedies like castor oil. Engage with communities online and offline that share your passion for holistic wellness. Sharing experiences and tips can provide additional insights and inspiration, enriching your journey.

Resources and Communities for Further Learning offer avenues for deepening your understanding and expanding your knowledge. Look for books, scientific studies, and workshops that delve into the science of natural remedies and their application. Online forums and social media groups focused on natural beauty and holistic health can be invaluable resources, offering support and a platform to exchange ideas.

As you continue to explore and integrate castor oil into your life, remember that the journey to natural beauty and wellness is deeply personal. What works for one person may not work for another, so listen to your body and adjust your practices accordingly. The goal is not perfection but progress towards a healthier, more radiant you, empowered by the knowledge and practices shared in this guide.

In embracing castor oil's natural benefits, you're not only taking steps towards enhancing your own health and beauty but also contributing to a more sustainable and environmentally conscious world. By choosing natural, time-honored remedies, you're part of a movement that values wellness, sustainability, and the power of nature's gifts.

Building Your Castor Oil Beauty and Wellness Routine

To seamlessly integrate castor oil into your beauty and wellness routine, begin by identifying specific areas of your health and beauty regimen that could benefit from its natural, healing properties. Castor oil, with its rich content of ricinoleic acid and omega-9 fatty acids, offers a versatile solution for a wide range of concerns. Here's a step-by-step guide to making castor oil a cornerstone of your daily self-care practices.

Step 1: Start with a Simple Patch Test

Before incorporating castor oil into your routine, conduct a patch test to ensure you don't have any allergic reactions. Apply a small amount of oil to a discreet area of your skin and wait for 24 hours. If there's no adverse reaction, you're ready to proceed.

Step 2: Incorporate into Your Skincare Routine

- Moisturizing: Use castor oil as a natural moisturizer by applying a few drops to your face and neck before bedtime. Its thick consistency deeply hydrates and locks in moisture.

- Cleansing: Try the oil cleansing method by massaging castor oil into your skin to dissolve impurities and makeup, then wash off with a warm, damp cloth.

- Acne Treatment: Due to its antimicrobial properties, castor oil can be dabbed on acne-prone areas to help reduce breakouts.

Step 3: Enhance Your Hair Care Regimen

- Scalp Treatment: Massage castor oil into your scalp to stimulate hair growth and control dandruff. Its anti-inflammatory properties soothe the scalp and support healthy hair follicles.

- Conditioner: Apply castor oil to the ends of your hair as a deep conditioner or use it as a base for homemade hair masks to restore shine and strength to your locks.

Step 4: Explore Its Wellness Applications

- Castor Oil Packs: For detoxification and pain relief, soak a piece of wool flannel in castor oil and place it on your abdomen. Cover with plastic wrap and a heating pad for 30-60 minutes.

- Joint and Muscle Relief: Rub castor oil directly onto sore joints or muscles to alleviate pain and inflammation, benefiting from its natural analgesic properties.

Step 5: Adopt Castor Oil for General Well-being

- Digestive Health: Consult with a healthcare provider about using castor oil packs for digestive issues. Its anti-inflammatory effects can be beneficial for conditions like IBS and bloating.

- Immune Support: Regular use of castor oil packs may also bolster your immune system by supporting lymphatic drainage and detoxification.

Step 6: Personalize Your Routine

Tailor the use of castor oil to your specific needs and preferences. Experiment with different applications, from skincare and haircare to general wellness, and adjust quantities and frequency based on your personal experience and the results you observe.

Step 7: Maintain Consistency

For best results, make castor oil a consistent part of your daily or weekly routines. Whether it's through topical application, hair treatments, or wellness practices, regular use maximizes the benefits of castor oil, contributing to your overall health and beauty.

By following these steps, you can build a comprehensive castor oil beauty and wellness routine that nurtures your body naturally. Embrace the journey of discovering how this ancient oil can transform your self-care practices, leading to radiant skin, lustrous hair, and a balanced, healthy body.

Continuing Your Journey Towards Radiant Health and Timeless Beauty

Embrace the evolving landscape of natural health and beauty, recognizing that your journey with castor oil is a dynamic process of learning, experimenting, and adapting. As you delve deeper into the myriad uses of this versatile oil, consider these strategies to enhance your exploration and application of castor oil for radiant health and timeless beauty.

- Expand Your Knowledge Base: Continuously seek out new research, books, and articles on the benefits and uses of castor oil. Science and holistic health fields are always advancing, offering fresh insights and innovative applications that can enrich your understanding and use of castor oil.

- Experiment with Customization: Personalize your castor oil remedies and treatments. Mix castor oil with other natural ingredients to create bespoke beauty products tailored to your skin and hair type. Adjust proportions based on your observations and results, fine-tuning your creations to meet your specific needs.

- Engage with a Community: Join forums, social media groups, or local workshops focused on natural remedies and holistic health. Sharing your experiences and learning from others can provide valuable support, inspiration, and new ideas for incorporating castor oil into your wellness routine.

- Practice Mindful Application: As you integrate castor oil into your daily practices, do so with intention and mindfulness. Pay attention to how your body responds to different applications, whether it's a castor oil pack for detoxification or a hair treatment for growth and strength. This mindful approach ensures you're not just going through the motions but truly connecting with your body's needs and responses.

- Sustain Ethical and Sustainable Choices: Source your castor oil and any additional ingredients from ethical, sustainable sources. Supporting companies that prioritize environmental stewardship and fair labor practices contributes to the well-being of the planet and communities, aligning with the holistic values at the heart of natural beauty and health.

- Document Your Journey: Keep a journal of your experiences, noting the formulations you try, the frequency of applications, and the outcomes you observe. This record not only tracks your progress but also serves as a valuable reference as you refine your use of castor oil over time.

- Incorporate Holistic Wellness Practices: Remember, true beauty and health are holistic. Alongside your castor oil routines, incorporate practices that nourish your body, mind, and spirit. Balanced nutrition, regular exercise, adequate rest, and stress-reducing activities like meditation or yoga complement the external applications of castor oil, enhancing your overall well-being.

- Stay Open to Evolution: Your needs and responses to castor oil treatments may change over time due to factors like aging, environmental changes, and shifts in your health. Stay open to adjusting your routines, exploring new uses for castor oil, and revisiting treatments you may have set aside.

By adopting these strategies, you ensure that your journey with castor oil is not just about maintaining beauty and health but about embracing a lifestyle that values natural remedies, personal well-being, and environmental consciousness. Continue to explore, learn, and grow in your natural beauty journey, letting castor oil be a key companion on your path towards radiant health and timeless beauty.

Resources and Communities for Further Learning

Exploring the vast world of natural health and beauty, especially the multifaceted uses of castor oil, is an enriching journey that extends beyond the pages of this guide. To deepen your understanding and application of castor oil in your daily life, a wealth of resources and communities are available at your fingertips. Here are some avenues to further your learning and connect with like-minded individuals who share your passion for holistic wellness.

- Online Forums and Social Media Groups: Platforms like Reddit and Facebook host numerous groups dedicated to natural remedies, holistic health, and DIY beauty. Search for groups focused on castor oil or broader topics like natural skincare and haircare. These communities are invaluable for sharing experiences, asking questions, and discovering new uses of castor oil.

- Blogs and Websites: Many bloggers and wellness influencers share their insights and experiments with castor oil. Websites like Wellness Mama and Earth Clinic feature articles, user testimonials, and DIY recipes that highlight castor oil's versatility. Bookmark these sites for easy access to a treasure trove of information.

- Workshops and Webinars: Keep an eye out for local and online workshops or webinars hosted by natural health practitioners and herbalists. These sessions can provide hands-on experience and direct learning from experts in the field. They often cover a range of topics, from making your own castor oil packs to integrating castor oil into holistic beauty routines.

- Books and Publications: While this guide serves as a comprehensive introduction, numerous books delve into the science and history of castor oil, as well as its practical applications. Look for titles by authors who specialize in natural health and herbal medicine. Your local library or bookstore's health and wellness section is a great place to start.

- YouTube Channels: Visual learners will appreciate the wealth of video content available on YouTube. Channels dedicated to natural health and beauty often feature tutorials on creating castor oil remedies, reviews of castor oil products, and tips for incorporating the oil into your wellness practices.

- Podcasts: For those who enjoy learning on the go, podcasts offer a convenient way to absorb information. Search for episodes focusing on natural remedies, holistic health, or personal wellness journeys. Podcasts can be a great source of inspiration and motivation as you explore the benefits of castor oil.

- Academic Journals and Research Papers: For a more scientific perspective, academic databases like PubMed offer access to research studies on castor oil. These papers can provide deeper insights into the oil's chemical properties, health benefits, and potential applications in medicine and skincare.

By engaging with these resources and communities, you'll not only expand your knowledge of castor oil but also connect with a supportive network of individuals who share your commitment to natural health and beauty. This journey of learning and discovery is ongoing, with each step offering new opportunities to enhance your wellness practices and enrich your life with the ancient wisdom of castor oil.

Download Your Fantastic Bonus Scanning This QR Code or Follow This Link:

[https://book-bonus.com/the-castor-oil-bible]

BONUS 1: The Castor Oil Manifesto: 120 Recipes for Natural Wellness
Unlock the secrets to optimal health with 120 transformative castor oil recipes—from revitalizing beauty treatments to healing home remedies.

BONUS 2: Unleash Nature's Secret: Boost Your Immunity and Ease Pain Naturally
Discover the potent benefits of castor oil for boosting your immune system and relieving pain with easy, natural solutions.

BONUS 3: Harmonize Your Hormones: Discover Natural Fertility and Wellbeing Solutions
Gain control over your hormonal health and fertility through the natural, balancing power of castor oil.

BONUS 4: Family Health Redefined: Gentle Remedies for Lifelong Vitality
Ensure your family's health and vitality with gentle, effective castor oil remedies that are safe for all ages.

BONUS 5: The Miracle Oil: Transform Your Health, Home, and Beauty Routine
Revolutionize your lifestyle with castor oil's diverse uses, enhancing not just your health but also your home and beauty routines.

DISCLAIMER

This book is intended solely for informational and educational purposes and should not be construed as medical, legal, or professional advice. The content within The Castor Oil Bible is based on the author's personal experiences and research, and while every effort has been made to ensure accuracy, Anita J. Batchelor, the publisher, and any associated entities make no representations or warranties of any kind with respect to the completeness or accuracy of the contents herein.

General Disclaimer:
Not Medical Advice: The information presented in this book is not intended to diagnose, treat, cure, or prevent any medical condition. It is not a substitute for professional medical advice, diagnosis, or treatment. Always consult a qualified healthcare provider before beginning any new health regimen, including those involving castor oil, natural remedies, or changes in diet.
Assumption of Risk: By reading this book, you acknowledge that the use of any remedies, treatments, or suggestions outlined herein is at your own risk. Anita J. Batchelor and the publisher disclaim any liability for injuries or adverse effects resulting directly or indirectly from the use or application of the information contained in this book.

Specific Risks Include but Are Not Limited To:
Allergic Reactions: Some individuals may be allergic to castor oil or other natural ingredients mentioned in this book. Test for allergies by applying a small amount to the skin before using.
Improper Application: Misuse of castor oil packs or ingestion of castor oil can lead to irritation, digestive upset, or more severe health issues.
Interactions with Medications: Certain natural remedies may interact with prescription medications. Always consult with a healthcare provider before combining natural remedies with prescribed treatments.
Exacerbation of Existing Conditions: Applying treatments in this book without proper medical guidance may worsen pre-existing skin conditions, digestive disorders, or other health issues.
Indemnification and Hold Harmless Clause:
By purchasing and/or reading The Castor Oil Bible, you agree to indemnify, defend, and hold harmless Anita J. Batchelor, the publisher, and any associated entities from and against any claims, damages, losses, liabilities, costs, or expenses (including reasonable attorneys' fees and costs) arising out of or in connection with your use or misuse of the information provided in this book.

By reading this book, you acknowledge that you have read, understood, and agreed to the terms of this disclaimer.